THE
BOOK
OF
CHAD

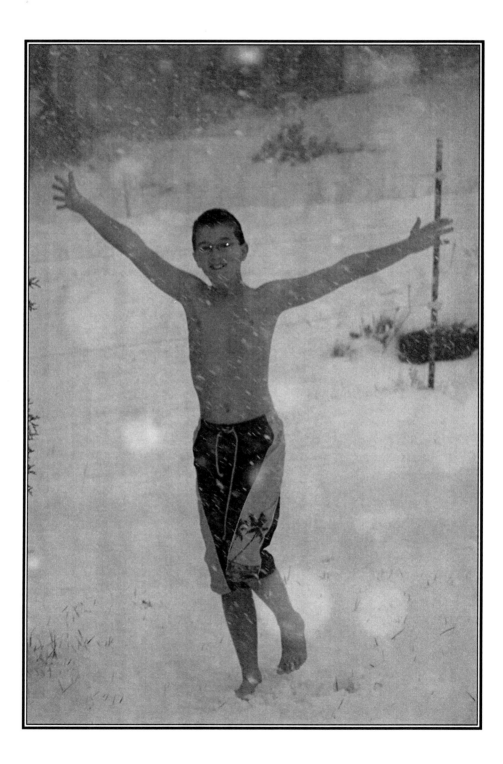

THE
BOOK
OF
CHAD

Richard Kozar

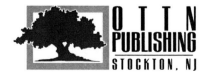
OTIN
PUBLISHING
STOCKTON, NJ

Frontispiece: Chad was complaining about being hot, so he went out in the snow wearing his swimsuit to cool down.

OTTN Publishing
16 Risler Street
Stockton NJ 08559
www.ottnpublishing.com

CPISA compliance information: Batch#080110.
For further information, contact OTTN Publishing, 609-397-4005.

First printing

1 3 5 7 9 8 6 4 2

Library of Congress Cataloging-in-Publication Data

Kozar, Richard.
  The book of Chad / by Richard Kozar.
    p. cm.
  Summary: "Tells the story of twelve-year-old Chad Scanlon and his battle against brain cancer"—Provided by publisher.
  ISBN 978-1-59556-038-4
  1. Scanlon, Chad—Health. 2. Brain—Cancer—Patients—Pennsylvania—Pittsburgh—Biography. 3. Cancer in children—Patients—Pennsylvania—Pittsburgh—Biography. I. Title.
  RC280.B7K69 2010
  616.99'4810092—dc22
  [B]
                                        2009050908

Cover photo courtesy Dolphin Quest, Inc., www.dolphinquest.com.

Author's Note: All of the people, places, and institutions featured in this book are real. However, since Chad's parents Marie-Paule and Jim relied on their best recollections of who said what, and when, in recounting their son's illness, we decided to rely on fictitious names for everyone but them, their daughter Sasha, and myself.

Table of Contents

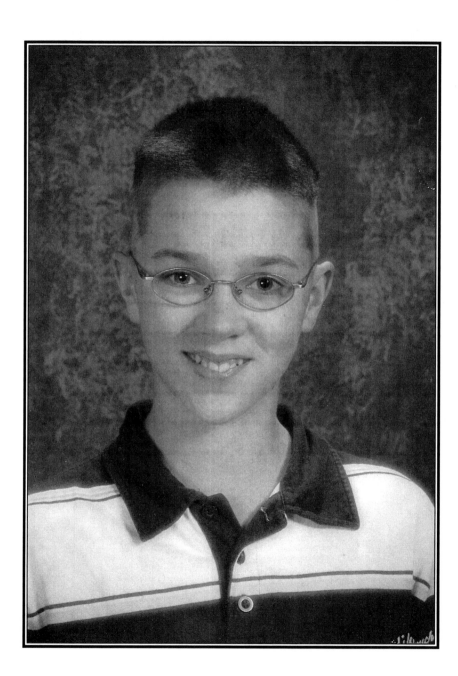

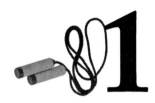

Calm Before Storm

I drove down the long gravel driveway to my friends' house, parked, and got out just in time for the trailing dust plume to envelop me. Live music filled the air as well—sad strains from a fiddle, filtering through the bedroom window and out into the yard. Accompanying it were chords from an acoustic guitar, with an electric keyboard in the background.

A handful of people sitting and chatting on the house's front porch were basking in the music and the afternoon sun on the cloudless May day. I waved to everyone in general but spoke only to one.

"How's Chad doing today, Abby?" I said to his aunt.

"The same. Go on back and say hi."

I entered the house, slipped off my leather boots, and walked the oak floors to the farthest bedroom, where I peered inside.

So these were the three minstrels I'd heard about. *A bearded country trio in blue jeans.* Each caught my eye in turn but continued to play. I was pretty sure the tune was Red River Valley.

My friend James Thomas Scanlon—known to us all as J.T.— sat on the right side of Chad's hospital bed. He was coaxing liquid from an eyedropper into his son's lips, which were cracked and dry. Chad's eyes were closed, but presumably he could hear the music. It would have been virtually impossible not to in the confines of this improvised concert hall.

J.T.'s wife, Marie-Paule, sat on Chad's left, tenderly holding his hand. She looked at me and managed a half smile, then wiped her son's forehead with a damp cloth. His younger sister Sasha was lying on a nearby bed, doing her homework.

As I contemplated the scene, J.T. maintained his drip regimen, so gently he could have been feeding a chick. Even so, Chad occasionally choked.

Their only son was tall for a 12 year old. However, his lanky frame seemed determined to slide, inch by inch, down the elevated bed, and his head threatened to roll off his pillow.

J.T. spotted me for the first time. He waited for the instrumentals to end before making introductions.

The music eventually stopped. "Guys, this is my buddy, Rich. That's Jeff on fiddle, Ray on guitar, and—I'm sorry, what's your name again?"

"Bill—"

"Bill playing the keyboard."

We all shook hands.

"I missed your performance the other day, and wasn't about to make the same mistake twice," I said. "I could hear your music outside. You guys are good."

"Much appreciated," Ray said. "We're all related, but none of us can read a lick of music." He turned to the center of everyone's attention. "But we're doing okay, right, Chad?"

He didn't respond.

"Okay, folks, what do you want to hear next?" Ray asked.

I struggled to think of a bluegrass song. "How about Orange Blossom Special?"

"I *do not* play Orange Blossom Special," the fiddler replied. He grinned, but I took him at his word.

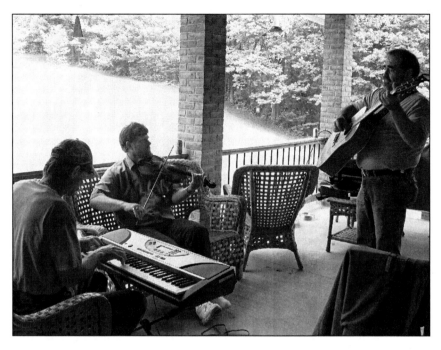

The trio of musicians playing bluegrass for Chad in spring 2007.

"Well, how about Tennessee Waltz?"

"Chad, is that okay with you?" Ray asked.

Chad squeezed Marie-Paule's hand almost imperceptibly.

"He says 'yes,'" she said.

"Good," said Ray. "Start us off, Jeff, and we'll join in after we hear the melody."

When the trio began harmonizing again, I realized the music was a perfect counterweight to the gloom that might otherwise have suffocated the room. I tried to conjure up a word that captured the setting, and settled on poignant.

I studied Chad's serene face, watched his shallow breaths, and tried to picture him as he was before. In situations like this there is always a before. Not so long ago, Chad had been on the cusp of adolescence, abundantly curious about the world and his future years in it. Now his future could be measured in days.

I swallowed hard, remembering my admonition to my

own college-age daughters when this ordeal had begun. "The last thing the Scanlons need is our tears. There will be plenty of time for tears."

Less than a year earlier, I had been driving home from a Saturday morning run when my cell phone rang. It was my wife, Elizabeth, calling to tell me J.T. had phoned from Children's Hospital in Pittsburgh. There weren't many details. All J.T. had said was Chad had been healthy the day before and was now gravely ill. "They just wanted us to know," Elizabeth said, and began crying.

I drifted back to that day. July 21, 2006, began with the promise of a celebration at the Scanlon house, which, after two years of hard work, was nearing completion. J.T. had built it from the ground up practically with his own hands, assisted from time to time by brothers and friends who had the skill, and inclination, to lend their own hands. One of the only tasks left to complete was installing porch railing, and not purely because of aesthetics. It just wouldn't do to have one of the guests coming to the evening's surprise bridal shower accidentally slip off the elevated concrete porch and land with a thud on the unseeded lawn. It wouldn't do at all.

As luck would have it, J.T. was temporarily on leave from his lineman's job. A week earlier, he had been helping move an upright freezer from the house of someone he barely knew. He had slipped while carrying it and bruised his ribs. That ruled out safely working on high-voltage power lines—but not hanging porch railing.

"It would be nice if the railing could be up tonight," Marie-Paule mentioned in the morning. "And," by the way, "it would be nice if Chad helped you."

At that moment, her son was lying on the spare couch they'd moved onto the front porch. He was reading *Harry Potter and the Goblet of Fire*.

"Chad," she said, "your dad needs help with the porch

railing. Why don't you work with him on it? You'll learn how he measures, cuts the pieces, and puts everything together."

He looked up from his book and frowned. "Do I have to?"

"Do it for Aurora. We want her to have a nice bridal shower, right?"

"Okaaaay."

He put down the book and said, "What time's the party tonight?"

"Seven. But you have jump rope practice at two, and then we have to come back and decorate the house for the party."

"The kids are going swimming to Ligonier pool after practice," he said. "Everybody on the team's going."

"Tonight is special here, too . . . Ariel's coming."

"She is?"

"Yes, Chad. I'm going to pick her up this morning."

"Good."

Ariel was Aurora Valdez's daughter from her first marriage. She had inherited her mother's deep tan and dazzling smile. She was a year older than Chad, but that hadn't stopped her from passing notes to him in the hallway at school. The shower was for her mother, who was marrying a Scanlon cousin.

J.T. walked onto the porch carrying his tool belt and drill. "Okay, Chad, let's get going on this railing."

Chad gave his mother a hug. "Is Sasha going with you to get Ariel?"

"Uh huh."

At that moment, his younger sister walked out of the house and stuck out her tongue at Chad.

"Mom!"

"We'll be back in an hour, Chad." Marie-Paule kissed him on the forehead. "Let's go, Sasha. And when we get back, we're going to clean house a while."

Now it was her turn to protest. ""Mom!"

Marie-Paule looked at her husband and added, "Have fun, guys."

J.T. reciprocated the look. "Okay, Chad. The first thing we need to do is measure the distance between the porch columns. Get my tape, buddy."

He continued, "Grab the end and hold it right next to the corner of the brick."

"Like this?"

"Yeah, that's good. . . I get twelve feet, three inches. Sound right?"

"If you say so."

"Okay, tell me how many inches are in twelve feet."

"I don't know."

"Well, how many inches are in a foot?"

"Twelve—"

"So multiply twelve times twelve."

"I don't have a calculator."

"Write it down on that piece of cardboard with a pencil and do it the old-fashioned way."

He watched his son scribble in the figures and do the math. "I get 144 inches," Chad said.

"Good. So we know we need to cut the railing down to 144 inches."

"One hundred forty seven, Dad. It's twelve feet, three inches, remember?"

J.T. looked at him and smiled. "See why I need you, Chad?"

He then laid the railing on the porch deck, measured and marked it with the pencil tucked behind his ear. He said, "What's the old saying?"

"Measure twice and cut once."

"Are we having fun yet?"

"One of us is."

J.T. laughed. "Wait till it's up. You can tell Ariel you helped hang it."

"I don't think she'll be very impressed."

"You never know, Chad. I didn't think anything I did in the Air Force was very impressive, and your mom married me."

"Oh, Dad."

They cut the railing, supported it on temporary blocks, and J.T. marked the holes where the metal support brackets would hang. He drilled the holes one by one and then ratcheted the bolts into place. When he was done, he said, "Not bad, Chad. It only took us an hour to hang the first section . . . just four more to go."

Chad was listening, and nodded, but his thoughts were elsewhere. In his daydream, he was already at jump rope practice that afternoon. His team at Holy Trinity School was supposed to put on a demonstration at the Ligonier Town Hall tomorrow. And a week later, he and several of his teammates would compete at nationals, which were scheduled for Hampton, Virginia.

"Chad . . . Chad!"

"What Dad?"

"I need you to hold the tape, buddy."

"Sorry. I was just thinking about jump rope."

J.T. didn't answer immediately. "You like jumping rope, don't you?"

"I love it."

His father marked the railing with his pencil. "You don't mind being the only boy on the team?"

"Nope. I don't care what people think. I like jumping rope. It's great exercise."

"Right . . . Can you put the end of the tape on the railing, bud?"

Chad did.

"You're really excited about going to nationals."

"Uh huh."

"What's your PR in speed?"

"Two-hundred ninety eight revolutions per minute."

His dad shook his head in amazement.

"Steady the railing while I cut it, okay?"

"Yep."

An hour later, Marie-Paule returned from picking up Ariel. As she walked up the sidewalk, she said, "Okay, that railing really looks nice, guys. Don't you think, Ariel?"

Chad's friend smiled and nodded.

"Hi, Ariel."

"Hi, Chad."

"Okay, girls, time to clean house," Marie-Paule said.

"I'd rather help dad," Sasha said.

"I know. But your dad already has a helper." The three went into the house.

Chad and J.T. continued their railing project. At one point, Chad said, "You really like doing this kind of work, don't you, Dad?"

"I love it."

"I can see why. You're really good at it. The railing's strong and looks nice."

His father nodded. "You're a big help."

"If you say so . . . but I think Sasha would rather be out here. She likes building things as much as you."

"Maybe . . . but she's not as good at math as you."

They both laughed.

Later, Marie-Paule came onto the porch carrying a tray with sandwiches and glasses of freshly squeezed lemonade. "Time for a break, boys."

"What time is it, mom?" Chad asked.

"One o'clock."

He looked at his dad while they ate. "I don't think we're going to finish it before I have to leave."

"That's okay. I'll keep at it while you're at jump rope."

"You sure?"

"Positive."

After lunch, Chad darted into the house and changed into shorts and a school T-shirt. He remembered to grab a towel on the way out.

He said goodbye to his father and waited in the family's Ford Expedition until his mother and the girls joined him.

Marie-Paule stepped onto the porch and said, "J.T., we'll be back around five." They kissed each other lightly on the cheek.

When she climbed into the SUV and buckled her belt, she said, "How did it go working with your dad?"

"Fine."

"No problems?"

"Nope . . . Mom, can we get going? I don't want to be late."

"Are you nervous, Chad?"

"A little . . . I just want to do well next week when we go to nationals."

"How do you feel?"

"Great."

"Then you'll do great, honey."

They drove up their gravel driveway until it intersected Ridge Road. They lived half an hour in any direction from the gas stations, grocery stores and populated towns surrounding Chestnut Ridge. The Scanlons loved the remoteness, but it did add miles and time to their inevitable trips off the mountain. As far as they were concerned, however, the solitude was worth the inconveniences.

Once in Ligonier, Chad said, "Mom, you know we're practicing in the basement of the Presbyterian church, right?"

"Yes, Chad, I know."

She pulled into a parking space at the church. Chad bounded out of the SUV before she put the vehicle in park. He ran to catch up to several of his teammates on their way into the building. Marie-Paule was locking the car when she heard a voice say, "He's raring to go, isn't he?"

Marie-Paule turned to the team's coach, Melissa Brandon, and replied, "He's been waiting to come all day."

"Good. The kids are in for a workout, though. The competition's going to be tough next week in Virginia."

"That's okay. Chad seems to have energy to burn today, Melissa."

The two women and girls walked into the basement, where the coach announced, "Okay, kids. Let's go through our stretching and warm-up exercises. I don't want anyone getting hurt today."

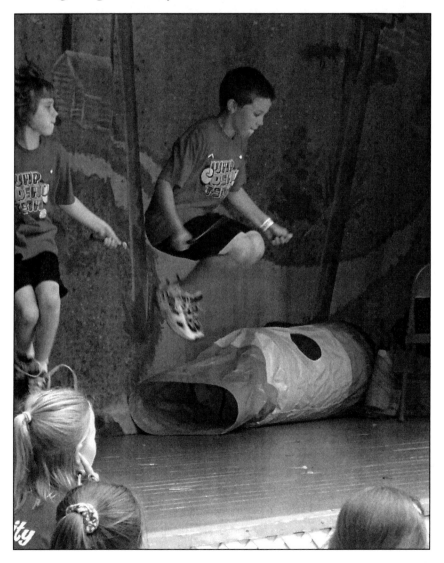

"Air Chad."

The team subsequently broke off into smaller groups to perform drills, which, for the next two hours, got progressively harder and faster. By the practice's conclusion, the youngsters and teens were breathless and sweating.

Nevertheless, Chad managed a smile when he walked over to his mother. "That was a workout," she said.

"Sure was." He changed the subject. "Mom, the other kids really want me to go swimming with them."

"Are you forgetting about Ariel and Aurora, and the party, Chad?"

"No . . . I just feel like I'm missing out."

"There'll be other days to swim."

"I guess."

She wrapped an arm around his shoulder and walked up the basement stairs. The sunlight that had brightened the day was now obscured by clouds, which were thickening and darkening from the west. Marie-Paule felt a large raindrop hit her head. "We've got to hurry, Chad. I need some things from the grocery store before we head home. Girls, time to run."

Before they reached the store minutes later, however, the rain had begun falling in earnest, and thunder rumbled in the distance. Chad, Ariel and Sasha decided to sit in the car while his mother shopped. A half hour later, she ran back to the Expedition, getting soaked in the process. "See Chad? Not a very good night for a swim."

"Or a bridal shower, mom."

"At least it's inside. Not even rain can ruin the party."

Marie-Paule looked at her watch. She decided to avoid the more scenic country roads on the way home. It would be 5:30 before they made it back, and there were still decorations to hang.

She looked at Chad. "I hope Dad's finished hanging the railing."

"Why?"

"Because we still have food to make, garland to hang,

and we all need showers."

He smiled. "I hope our well holds out."

"Don't even joke about that, Chad."

By the time they pulled next to their house, the rain had stopped, and the skies partially cleared. Marie-Paule saw her husband had been busy while they were away. "You only have one more section of railing to do," she said.

"I don't know if I'll finish in time, though," J.T. replied. "I still have to clean up the porch and myself."

"Yes, and the girls and I still have cleaning to do and decorations to hang."

As she and her son piled grocery bags on the kitchen island, Marie-Paule thought about all the tasks remaining before the party.

She turned to Sasha, "Girls, at some point I'll need you to clean the bathrooms and wipe the floors."

"Aw, Mommmm."

"Or you could start hanging the garland, while I start making the hors d'oeuvres." She continued, "Chad, you're taller than Ariel. Help them, would you?"

"Okay," he said with a sigh.

"Are you tired, honey?"

"A little. I think I'm getting a headache."

"Drink lots of water. You're probably dehydrated."

Marie-Paule emptied vegetables out of the grocery bags and rinsed them in the sink. She pulled out a party tray and began arranging the broccoli, carrots and cauliflower on it. She could overhear the children talking.

"You looked great in practice, Chad," Ariel said.

"Thanks."

"How do you think you'll do at nationals?"

He shrugged as he held up a strand of garland for taping. He realized as he did that he could smell his own body odor. He dropped his arm as quickly as he could, but if Ariel was offended, she didn't let on. She, on the other hand, smelled wonderful. Not of perfume, but a milder scent that reminded him of lemons. She caught him looking at her. "What?"

He blushed. "Nothing."

Sasha giggled. "Do you want me to leave?"

Marie-Paule smiled without looking up. All she had remaining to do was arrange another tray with fruit and one with rolled tortellini appetizers. She normally preferred to make her own hors d'oeuvres, but Sam's Club was hard to beat and she was pressed for time.

By six p.m., her work was done, and she realized she had less than an hour to shower. She was washing her hands when she saw two cars pulling down the driveway. She recognized the occupants as J.T.'s Aunt Tessie and her daughter Chris. Tessie's son Kevin was Aurora's fiancé.

"Sasha, I have to shower," she said. "Aunt Tessie is here with Chris. When you're done with the garland, help them with their food, would you?"

"Okay."

Marie-Paule noticed Chad had slumped in a chair. "Tired, honey?"

He nodded. "My head hurts."

"Keep drinking water, sweetheart. You've had a long day."

He didn't answer.

Marie-Paule walked down the hallway to her bedroom just before Tessie and Chris came in carrying Tupperware containers and bags of snacks. They placed them on the counter, greeted Ariel and Sasha, and set to work.

J.T. came in five minutes later, sweaty and covered with grime. "Hey, Aunt Tessie." He gave her a hug. "How're you doing, Chris?"

"Great . . . J.T., the railing looks beautiful."

"I hope it holds everyone up," he said, "or Marie-Paule will push me off the porch tonight."

He was about to head for his bedroom when he saw Chad get up slowly from a lounge chair and shuffle to his room. J.T. washed his hands quickly in the kitchen sink and followed. When he entered his son's room, he saw him lying on his bed. "Chad, what's wrong, buddy?"

"My head hurts, dad."

J.T. knew Chad was no stranger to headaches. "You want a neck rub, pal?" That usually did the trick.

"No."

"Okay, I'll send mom to see you in a couple minutes."

He walked into his own bedroom and heard the shower door open in the bathroom. He tapped on the bathroom door and stuck his head in. "Marie-Paule?"

"Uhhh, I'm not dressed yet."

"So I see."

"What do you want, J.T.?"

"Chad says his head hurts. You should probably check on him when you're dressed."

"What time is it?"

"A little after six . . . Why?"

"Oh, because everyone'll be here in another half hour, and I have to dry my hair, put on my make-up—"

"You look great just the way you are."

"You're the only one who'll think so . . . Now is Chad really sick, or just being Chad?"

"I don't know. I'm no doctor."

She didn't disagree. "All right. Now go away, s'il vous plait."

He grinned and shut the door. While he was undressing, his wife came out and slipped into a pink summer dress he hadn't seen before. "Is that new?"

"Yes, dear. I want tonight to be special."

He thought a moment. "What's Sasha wearing?"

"Not her new dress. I told her this morning it's for the wedding." She was looking for her shoes when her husband said, "Aunt Tessie and Chris are here."

"Good. I need all the help I can get."

"You're doing great."

"I'll be doing great when my hair is dried and I put my

eyes on."

"Mom!"

She walked out of her bedroom. "Coming, Chad."

She was surprised to find him in bed. "What's wrong, honey? Daddy says you have a headache."

"My head really hurts, Mom."

"Well, do you want an aspirin? What do you want me to do, honey?"

"Mom, I need *help*!"

Just then, Marie-Paule heard her daughter say, "Mom, Aunt Tina's here."

Thank God.

She went out onto the porch to greet J.T.'s aunt, who had been a paramedic once upon a time.

"Hi, Aunt Tina," she said.

"How's it going, Marie-Paule? Is everything coming along?"

"Sort of—"

"What?"

"Chad's not feeling well—"

"Really?"

"Yes, he says his head really, really hurts. Could you check on him?"

"Sure, sweetie."

The two came into the house and immediately went into Chad's bedroom. Tina said softly, "Hello, Chad. Your mom says your head hurts. Mind if I take a look?"

He moaned but otherwise didn't respond.

Tina sat on the bed and looked into Chad's eyes. She didn't like what she saw. "Marie-Paule, find something we can put between Chad's teeth. A popsicle stick, a toothbrush, even a wash cloth."

"Why, what's wrong?"

"I think he's having a seizure . . . and you may want to call an ambulance."

J.T. stuck his head in the room. "Aunt Tina, did I hear

you say to call an ambulance?"

"Yes, J.T."

"Well, we can take Chad to the hospital."

"First we should get him onto the porch, J.T. He's burning up."

J.T. grabbed his son under his shoulders while his aunt hoisted Chad's legs. They didn't realize how heavy he was until they tried to lift him. "Marie-Paule, grab the door, would you?" her husband said.

In the few moments it took to carry him out of the house, Chad began shivering violently. They laid him on the porch couch and covered him with a surplus Army blanket. "I'll get the Expedition," J.T. said.

"No," Tina replied. "Call 9-1-1 and say you need an ambulance."

J.T. dialed as fast as he could.

"9-1-1 dispatch."

"Yeah, this is Jim Scanlon. I live on 401 Ridge Road. I need an ambulance for my son."

"What's the emergency, sir?"

"We think he's having a seizure."

"Is that location in Cook Township?"

"Yeah, about two miles east of Possum Hollow Road."

"I'm dispatching the nearest ambulance service, sir. They'll be there as soon as they can."

"Thanks."

Marie Paule tried to calm herself. *It's just dehydration. He's just been running around too much today.*

She pulled a chair up to her son and held his hand. It was cold and clammy. "He's going to be all okay, right Tina?"

She nodded gently.

Twenty minutes went by. Then thirty.

More cousins and friends had arrived, and were on the porch now, looking and listening for the sound of an approaching vehicle. "Good Lord, what's taking so long?" Tina whispered to no one in particular. She went back into

the house and called 9-1-1 on her cell phone. After the initial exchange of information, she said. "Where the hell's that
ambulance? We called over a half hour ago?"

"Sorry, m'am. The call went out to two ambulances in
closest proximity to your location, but both were handling
emergencies when they got the call . . . they're en route now."

She hung up without another word and went back onto
the porch. "I think they'll be here soon," she said.

Two minutes later, everyone heard the chug of diesel
engines coming down the drive. Two vehicles pulled near the
house, and three EMTs disembarked. There was a flurry of
activity around Chad as they checked his eyes, pulse and res-
piration.

"I think he's having some sort of seizure," Tina whispered
to one. "You need to get him to the hospital as soon as possible." He nodded.

They brought a gurney up to the porch and lifted Chad
onto it. J.T. turned to Marie-Paule and said, "You stay here
and handle the shower. I'll go with them."

"I don't *think* so."

"—Okay."

"Mom, I'm coming, too," Sasha said. Tears were rolling
down her cheeks.

Her mother turned to her and knelt down. "I don't think
that's necessary, honey—"

"But—"

"Someone has to run this party. I need you and Ariel to
help me," she explained. "You know what's going on, this big
secret for Aurora. You know what to do, you know where the
food is, you know what the games are . . . besides, I need
someone to finish decorating the house."

Sasha began sobbing uncontrollably.

"You know what, Sasha? If you want, you can go put on
the dress you got for Aurora's wedding."

Her daughter looked up at her. "Can I wear my new
shoes, too?"

"Certainement. Look pretty, sweetie, and take care of this shower for me. This is supposed to be a happy event."

"Okay . . . Call me, okay?"

"We will." She kissed her daughter's forehead, and left her with her female cousins, who had begun crying as well.

She hurried to catch up with the ambulance crew. "I'm riding with my son, yes?"

"Sorry, m'am," said an EMT. "I'll be in the back with him while my buddy drives. You can ride passenger in the second ambulance, though."

Marie-Paule nodded.

J.T. said to her, "Go ahead. I'll be driving right behind you." They gripped each other's hands a second and parted.

J.T. glanced at his watch as the motorcade pulled out. On a good day, he could be in downtown Latrobe in twenty-five minutes. *This is turning out to be anything but a good day.*

The caravan wound its way down the mountain at a brisk but not breakneck pace. Before long, it had reached Youngstown, the tiny village about five miles from Latrobe's Excela Hospital. The stop light in the lone intersection was red. Without warning, the lead ambulance hit its siren.

Marie-Paule turned to her driver. "Is that normal, or is something wrong?"

"No, we sometimes do that when we want to get through traffic," he replied. "It doesn't mean anything."

"Okay."

They sped off, covering the final miles of the trip in less than ten minutes. Marie-Paule began to breathe more evenly the moment she saw the hospital towering on the horizon. Before she knew it, the first ambulance was backing up to the Emergency Room entrance. By the time she gathered her purse, Chad's gurney was already being wheeled inside. She couldn't see J.T.'s Expedition. Presumably her husband was parking. She didn't wait.

Inside, one of the EMTs escorted her through Triage and down the hall to an examination room, where nurses and doctors swarmed around Chad. Marie-Paule watched in shock as a physician inserted a breathing tube down Chad's throat. A nurse noticed her distress and said, "I'm sorry, but you'll have to wait outside."

"He may be having some kind of seizure, my aunt said. She used to be a paramedic."

The nurse nodded. "We'll let you know as soon as we learn something."

Marie-Paule's head was spinning. She sat down in the nearest hallway chair before she fell down. *He didn't drink enough today. He's just dehydrated.*

A short time later, a woman in a white coat approached her. "Are you Mrs. Scanlon?"

"Yes."

The woman held out her hand. "I'm Tracy Holdorfer. I'm sending Chad for a CAT scan. They'll be bringing him back from radiology in a little while." Marie-Paule noticed the M.D. on her nametag.

"A CAT scan?" she asked.

"Yes, it'll give me a better picture of what's going on in his head." She gave a sympathetic smile. "You can stay here and I'll let you know when we have the results."

Time crawled while Marie-Paule waited anxiously for the CAT scan films. Eventually, she heard footsteps coming down the hall. "I have the results," Holdorfer told her. "I want to show you." Her voice was quiet, sweet.

Nevertheless, Marie-Paule felt a surge of anxiety. *Something is wrong. This is not dehydration. Wake up!*

The doctor hung the films on a nearby illuminated screen. She pointed to a shadow on the CAT scan. "See this here? This is bleeding."

Marie-Paule looked at her intently. "It's bad?"

"Yes, it is." Unexpectedly, the doctor hugged her. "I've already called Children's Hospital in Pittsburgh. Hopefully, a helicopter's going to be able to come . . . This is out of our hands. We stabilized him basically, but he needs to go."

J.T. walked up at that moment. He had been registering Chad for admission. After overhearing what the doctor had just said, he asked, "Why are you worried about the helicopter being able to come?"

"It's the weather. They can't fly during a thunderstorm . . . But let's hope for the best."

In a fortunate turn of events, the storms did calm. Twenty-five minutes later, a nurse approached Chad's parents. "The helicopter's going to be landing. We have to get Chad ready for the flight."

"Can I go with him?" Marie-Paule asked.

"Sorry, no. There isn't room . . . Have you ever been to Children's before?"

"No," they answered.

"All right. Sir, you should go get your car and bring it up the emergency room entrance. In the meantime, I'll send in an aide. He'll talk to your wife about how to get to Children's . . . good luck."

In a few minutes, a man in a lab coat came into the room and introduced himself. He said, "Here's a map for the drive to Pittsburgh, with directions from the Parkway to Children's Hospital. It should take just over an hour this time of night." He handed them to Marie-Paule.

"Now, do you have a credit card?"

"Yes."

"Do you need any cash?"

"No. I'm fine."

He nodded and came over to hug her. "God bless you."

Marie-Paule looked at the man. Although he had attempted to reassure her, he had done anything but.

Outside, the helicopter rose from the landing pad until it reached sufficient altitude, then pivoted to the west and sped toward Children's Hospital, a division of the University of Pittsburgh Medical Center's sprawling chain of health institutions.

J.T. was waiting at the emergency room entrance when

Marie-Paule came out. Neither said a word as he sped off.

Forty-five minutes later, they exited Pittsburgh's Parkway East at the Oakland exit—and promptly got lost.

Near panic, Marie-Paule called her sister, who she hoped was more familiar with the city. The first words out of her mouth were, "Elaine, Chad's had a stroke. They've flown him by helicopter to Children's Hospital in Pittsburgh, but J.T. and I can't find it." Her eyes were brimming with tears.

"A stroke? Marie-Paule, children don't get strokes. Children get aneurysms, which we have on both sides of our family." She paused, then added, "Where are you now?"

"Somewhere in Oakland, I think."

"I'm coming," Elaine said.

"No, you live too far away. Stay where you are . . . We just can't find the hospital."

"It's near the University of Pittsburgh, Marie-Paule."

"I know. I think we just missed a street somewhere."

Suddenly, J.T. said, "I know where we are. It's right up ahead."

"I've got to go, Elaine. I'll keep you informed. J.T. and I need to be together and figure out what's going to happen. We don't need any distractions. We're just going to have to deal with this ourselves tonight."

"Okay, Marie-Paule. Call me the minute you know anything."

The Scanlons pulled into Children's main entrance and were immediately directed to Chad's room in Intensive Care. When they opened the door, they found him lying unconscious on a bed. Marie-Paule felt her pulse racing as she assessed his situation. There was a tube attached to his skull, draining bloody fluid, by all appearances, from his brain. The ventilator tube was inserted into her son's throat, meaning a machine was still breathing for him. She reached for J.T.'s hand and gripped it tightly.

Within minutes the physician on duty joined them in the room. "Your son needs an MRI to determine what's causing

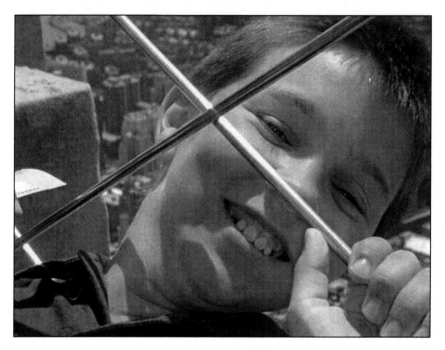

Chad hamming it up atop the Empire State Building before illness.

the bleed, but first we have to stabilize his vital signs for two hours," he said. "The MRI lab is in another section of the hospital, and Chad just isn't stable enough to be moved yet."

Marie-Paule nodded. "We can wait in here, though, yes?"

"Of course."

She sat down in a chair next to Chad's bed and looked at her watch. It was nearly eleven p.m. Back at her house, the shower should be winding down about now. She said to J.T., "I need to call the house. Somebody has to take Sasha home with them tonight."

She called on her cell phone. Sasha answered. "How's Chad, Mom?"

She explained the situation as gently as possible, but warned, "We're going to be here all night, at least. Can you go home with Aurora?"

"I guess."

"Okay, honey. Can I talk to Cindy?"

"Uh huh."

When her cousin came on she again explained Chad's condition, adding, "We're probably going to be here overnight. Sasha knows everything, but don't tell anyone else, especially Aurora, until the party's over. I don't want to spoil the shower."

"Absolutely. Anything else I can do?"

"Pray."

Cindy said, "I already am."

Marie-Paule hung up and pulled her chair next to Chad's bed to hold his hand. Her eyelids drooped, but she refused to surrender to sleep.

She sat there quietly for over an hour, hoping, praying, and remembering how vital Chad had been just that afternoon. It was too much to process in the span of one evening.

At some point, a nurse came into the room to check on Chad, and she immediately paged the attending physician. He rushed into the room, took one look at Chad's drain tube, and said, "Your son's having another bleed. I'm afraid you'll have to leave till we can stabilize him again. The nurse will show you the waiting room."

They were escorted down the hall to a drab room furnished with a single table for four, a cook-top range, and perhaps a dozen chairs. There was no artwork hung, no photographs. Six people were sitting in distinct pairs around the room. They looked up at the Scanlons with shell-shocked expressions that conveyed more than words.

Marie-Paule and J.T. sat down near one couple. Their son had been in an ATV accident, the mother explained after introductions. The surgeons had to remove part of his skull to accommodate the swelling in his brain. The skin had been temporarily pulled back over the damaged area. "They're keeping part of his forehead in a freezer," she confided in a whisper. "Can you imagine? Part of my little boy's head is in a freezer."

She pointed to another couple that rose to leave without

saying hello. "Their little boy's five, or six, I can't remember exactly. They mentioned he's blonde, like my boy," she said. "He was hit by a car this morning . . . they've spent every minute they can in his room."

Marie-Paule picked up a nearby magazine and was flipping through the pages when J.T. said, "Since when have you been a fan of Sports Illustrated?"

"I'm just trying to keep my mind off—"

"I know . . . I'm gonna lay back and try to get some sleep. It's going to be a long night."

She smiled wearily at him and went back to her magazine.

Marie-Paule was in mid-doze herself a half-hour later when she heard footsteps coming down the hall. She snapped to, only to hear them pass on by. This drill repeated itself several more times until, finally, at midnight, a doctor came in and introduced himself to them. He said his name, but it didn't even register. What did was when he mentioned he was an assistant to a neurosurgeon.

"We just completed an emergency MRI of Chad's head, and the results came back," he began. "We've got to operate. Your son has a tumor in his brain. It's very deep, and the operation is very sensitive because it's in a high-traffic area. In order to save Chad's life, we've got to go in right now. We've called in Dr. Benjamin Klein as the surgeon. He's quite capable. In fact, he's one of the best, world-renowned. Chad is probably in the best hands possible."

He continued, "There are some surgical consent forms you'll need to sign. I'll leave them with you. When you're done, pick up that phone over there and dial the nurse's station. They'll come pick them up . . . Everything clear?"

"Yeah," said J.T.

"This doctor—" Marie-Paule said.

"Dr. Klein—"

"Yes. Is he at the hospital?"

"No, Mrs. Scanlon. I imagine he's sleeping by now. But

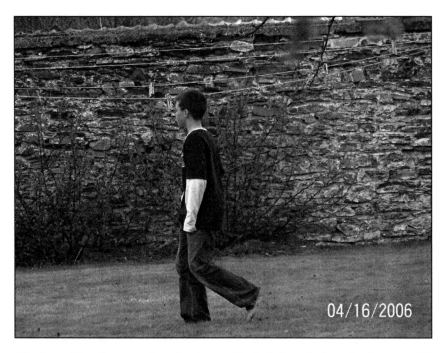

04/16/2006

Chad strolling in grandmother's yard in Belgium before he became ill.

we've paged him and he'll be here as soon as he can."

She nodded.

When the doctor left, Marie-Paule turned to her husband. "Are we doing the right thing signing for this surgery? We don't even know whether it's best for Chad. What if something goes wrong? . . . What if he's not the best doctor? . . . What will he be like after the surgery?"

J.T. thought a moment. "I think what the doctor told us, honey, is that Chad will die without the surgery. He'll just keep bleeding, and they have to do something to stop it." He squeezed her hand. "I don't think we have a choice."

"I know. I'm just so scared for him."

When the nurse came to retrieve the consent forms, Marie-Paule asked her, "How long will surgery last?"

"I can't say for sure, Mrs. Scanlon, but I would think at least several hours. Brain surgery is never easy."

She continued, "I'll ask someone to bring you updates as

often as they can, okay?"

"Yes. Thank you."

J.T. said, "We should try getting some sleep."

"I've been trying," she said. "Every time someone walks down the hallway, I think it's for us."

They both closed their eyes and slumped in their chairs.

The next thing J.T. knew, someone was tugging his shoulder. He looked up to see his brother, Blake, and their father, Chuck. "Hey, guys. What time is it? . . . What are you doing here?"

"We figured you could use a care package," Blake replied. He handed Marie-Paule a travel bag. She looked inside and began pulling out items. "Oh, look, J.T., underwear for you, pajamas for us both, toothbrushes, deodorant . . . and a bag of candy."

Blake grinned. "Not just any candy, Marie-Paule. Lifesavers. You always need lifesavers when you come to a hospital."

J.T. brought his family up to date on Chad's condition, including the surgery.

"How long has he been in?" Blake asked.

J.T. studied his watch. "About two hours. They had to call the surgeon in from home. I think it started around one a.m."

Blake looked around the room. "Not a very cheery place, is it?'

"No," Marie-Paule said. "And the families here . . . they are all so tense, so nervous . . ."

"And numb," J.T. added.

Blake and his father stayed in the waiting room for an hour or so, until J.T. said, "Go home, get some rest. We might need you later on today." And the two men left.

At five a.m. a tall, athletic man in surgical greens came into the waiting room. "Are you the Scanlons?" he said to them.

"Yes."

"Hi. I'm Benjamin Klein."

Marie-Paule began relaxing the second she saw him. The doctor had the bearing of a television surgeon. *This guy is somebody.*

He began, ""As you know, Chad has a tumor. I tried to remove as much of it as possible, but there was so much bleeding, it was a very challenging procedure."

Marie-Paule's heart sank, but she remained silent.

Klein continued, "Now we have to see what's going to happen. Chad will let us know what he can or can't do anymore. When you have brain surgery, you have to expect side effects. They might be motor skills, might be speech, but only Chad will let us know."

He added, "We'll also have to wait several days for the results of the biopsy."

The Scanlons didn't know how to respond.

"You can see Chad now. He's out of recovery, and back in his room in ICU."

"Thank you for all you've done," J.T. managed.

Klein shook his hand and left.

When Marie-Paule and her husband walked into Chad's room, they steadied themselves for what they might see. It didn't help. There were now two catheters draining fluid from his skull, and he was still attached to a breathing machine. He was also connected to more wires and devices than their home entertainment center, J.T. thought. With tears welling up in his eyes, he stifled the overpowering urge to turn around and flee the scene altogether.

Marie-Paule's reaction was just the opposite. Her son's dependence on machines made her heart ache. She was determined not to leave his side. She took up a vigil next to his bed.

Fifteen minutes later, J.T. said, "I can't take this anymore. I've got to get some air."

"It's okay," she said. "Go."

And so Saturday morning went, with Marie-Paule glued

to Chad's bedside, while his dad came and went as his emotions permitted. During a shift change between nurses, one said to Marie-Paule, "I'm sorry, but I need to bring the next shift nurse up to date on Chad's condition. It'll just take five minutes or so. You can wait outside, or get something to eat or drink in the cafeteria."

She could tell Marie-Paule was only leaving reluctantly. "Mrs. Scanlon, give me your cell phone number. If anything happens, I'll get in touch with you right away."

"Anything, good or bad, call me."

"I will."

The hours passed uneventfully, however.

At one point, J.T.'s cell phone rang. He glanced at the caller ID and realized who was calling. He answered and said, "Hey, Rich."

"Hey, Jimmy. Elizabeth told me you called about Chad. What's going on?"

"Well, he's got a tumor in his brain, and it started to bleed last night."

"Good Lord."

"Yeah. Anyway, we life-flighted him to Pittsburgh last night and they took him into surgery about one a.m. He didn't come out until five."

"How's he doing?"

"Well, the doctor says he came through it pretty well. He got some of the tumor out, but since there was so much bleeding, he can't be sure. Chad's still under heavy sedation, and we're just waiting for him to wake up, basically."

"What do you guys need, J.T.? I can come in whenever you need me."

"Thanks, man. But Marie-Paule's sister Elaine's coming in with her husband, Greg, and they're supposedly bringing plenty to eat. Maybe tomorrow or—hell—I don't even know what day it is."

"Still Saturday, bud." I tried to concentrate on my driving and the phone call. "Okay, I'll check back in with you tomorrow. And we'll keep all you guys in our prayers. Give Marie-Paule our love, would you?"

"I will. Thanks, brother, I appreciate your call."

Saturday turned into Sunday, and still Chad didn't wake. The one bright note came courtesy of Dr. Klein. He told the Scanlons, "Based on an MRI we took of Chad today, it looks like I did a better job removing the tumor than I expected to do." Even so, he again warned them that Chad could have any number of side effects from the surgery, including loss of speech or other motor skills.

On Monday, I drove to Pittsburgh for a visit. I found Marie-Paule and J.T. in the parent waiting room and gave them both hugs. They looked surprisingly well. "How's he doing?"

"No change, really," J.T. said. "Do you want to go see him?"

"You bet."

"C'mon."

We entered the Intensive Care Unit and proceeded to Chad's room. Nurses greeted J.T. with smiles along the way. "I see you've made fast friends with the female corps already, buddy," I said.

"You know me. Like to make myself at home."

We came to Chad's room and entered. I said, "Good grief, J.T., Chad looks taller than you lying there. I haven't paid enough attention to how much he's grown lately."

Chad's eyes were closed and he was breathing in perfect rhythm to the ventilator. Both of us watched him without saying a word.

Finally, I turned and said, "It's every parent's worst nightmare, isn't it?"

J.T.'s eyes glassed up. "It's tearing me up. I can only stand to be in here for a few minutes at a time."

I nodded and put my arm over his shoulder. "When my sister was sick, J.T., she always told me, 'One day at a time . . . that's the best advice I can give you."

He nodded.

"Come on, Jimmy. I want to spend some time with Marie-Paule, too."

I turned back to the bed and said, "Bye, Chad. Next time I see you I expect you'll be awake. Take care, buddy."

We walked back to the waiting room. I noticed a large family of what appeared to be farmers sitting around the room. They reminded me of the rural folk from Lancaster, Pennsylvania. J.T. whispered to me, "They're Amish. Their little boy has some kind of birth defect, I think . . . They're nice people."

I hugged Marie-Paule. "I have nothing wise to say, I'm afraid, other than you're in our prayers and thoughts."

She smiled through wet eyes. "It's hard, but hey, what are you gonna do?"

I greeted Elaine and her husband as well. "What have you guys brought that smells so good?"

"Stew," Elaine replied. "We're just about to eat. Sit with us, yes?"

I shook my head. "I don't need to eat right now, thanks. But you guys go right ahead."

The four of them sat down, said a quiet blessing, and began eating. Then J.T. abruptly stood and walked over to one of the older Amish men. I heard him say, "Would you folks like some stew? We've got plenty to go around."

The farmer looked to his wife, who nodded shyly, and then turned back to J.T. "Thank you, kindly. We would love to share your food with you." J.T. smiled and said, "We have plates and spoons. Come on over and help yourselves."

Soon ladles were clanging in the pot as young children stood in line with their elders to get a bowl of stew. Then, they returned to their seats and ate in silence.

I stayed over an hour watching everyone eat, talk and laugh, as if this were just another of the frequent picnics being held in the Scanlons' backyard. Finally, when the meal was finished and cleanup done, I stood. "Time to go, guys. Let's make with the goodbyes."

When I hugged Marie-Paule, I asked, "What do you need?"

"Nothing."

"Really? Think harder."

"Really, we have food . . . Elaine and Greg are here every day . . . "

"Okay, how about stuff from home, or a ride for anybody?"

She thought momentarily. "We're good for the time being."

"Okay. I won't call you guys, you just call me if you feel the need."

"Will do," said J.T.

I left, and was walking out of the hospital when I decided to call home. "Hello, Elizabeth."

"How are they doing?"

"Better than most people."

"Really?"

"Yeah. They're amazing."

"Why?"

"Oh, you know, laughing and joking over dinner, like they were back on the Ridge in their house."

"How's Chad?"

"Still sedated. It tears your heart out just looking at him hooked up to all those machines."

She didn't answer.

"You know the neatest thing, though?"

"What?"

"There was an Amish family in the waiting room. Elaine had brought in a big pot of stew, and they were all sitting down to eat . . ."

"And—"

"And J.T. gets up and asks the family if *they'd* like something to eat . . . His son is on a ventilator in intensive care, and he's worried whether these people would like something to eat."

Elizabeth was silent.

I collected myself for a few moments, then said, "I'm starting to think I believe in angels."

"The kind with wings?"

I laughed softly. "No, the kind walking among us down here."

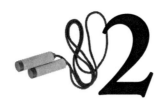

"J'ai froid"

Chad had remained in a coma for several days. Finally, late one night, when the Scanlons were trying to catch some sleep in the parents' waiting room, a nurse remembered Marie-Paule's insistence on being called with any news. Doctors had begun reducing the oxygen levels in Chad's ventilator tube to encourage him to breathe on his own, and he was fighting back—a hopeful sign. So she called her, despite the hour.

After the brief conversation, Marie-Paule woke J.T. to tell him.

"Honey, we need our sleep," he grumbled. "You can't keep asking them to call for every tiny thing Chad does."

"I'm sorry you feel that way . . . I need to know."

The following morning, a social worker came to meet with the Scanlons and introduced himself as Perry. "At some point you folks are going to meet Dr. Rachael Hemminger," he said.

"Why do we need another doctor?" asked Marie-Paule. "I like Dr. Klein just fine."

"Dr. Hemminger's a pediatric oncologist," Perry replied.

"Oh." Marie-Paule didn't know what to think. She hadn't even allowed herself to consider that her son may have a malignant tumor. In her mind, people with cancer were tired, weak, and lost weight, long before they were even diagnosed. *No,* she thought, *Chad can't have cancer. There's no point in meeting another doctor.*

Nevertheless, a day later Rachael Hemminger stopped by to visit Chad in ICU. She introduced herself and checked his chart. As quickly as she'd come in, she left, without ever discussing the tumor itself.

During her visit the following day, however, the Scanlons made a point of asking about the biopsy.

"I'm still awaiting definitive results," Hemminger said.

"Can you tell us at least whether it's benign or malignant?" Marie-Paule asked.

"Well, let's just wait."

J.T. persisted. "You know if it's bad or not. Can you at least tell us that?"

She hesitated. "Yes. It's malignant."

The morning after the cancer diagnosis, nurses asked the Scanlons to step out of Chad's room in the ICU during a routine shift change. "Go downstairs to the snack shop or grab breakfast in the cafeteria," they were told.

But first, J.T. decided to take a detour to a nearby restroom, where he couldn't help noticing a well-dressed, ruggedly built African American at the sink next to him. *This guy could be a Pittsburgh Steeler, except he's wearing a suit instead of black and gold.*

"How you doin'?" J.T. said.

"I'm doing fine. How are you doing?"

"Ohhh . . . I'm doin' fine, too."

The man stopped washing his hands and turned to J.T. "Son, your voice is telling me one thing but your eyes are telling me something different."

J.T. paused a moment, and sat himself on the counter. And then he began pouring out his soul to this total stranger, telling him of Chad's emergency surgery, being in a coma, and then the numbing news that his tumor was malignant. Finally, he said, "I'm sorry. My name's Jim Scanlon."

"Roger Jamison."

"Can I ask what you do here?"

"I'm the chaplain."

"No wonder you could tell I wasn't fine. . . Do you have an office here someplace?"

"I do."

"Would you mind meeting my wife? She's waiting in the hall, and I think we both need someone to talk to."

"Let's go."

Outside, before J.T. introduced Jamison to his wife, he said, "Hey, what do I call you—Reverend?"

"How about Roger."

"Okay. Marie-Paule? I've got someone here you should meet. Roger Jamison, this is Marie-Paule."

"Hello."

"Hi."

"You two know each other?" she asked with a smile, wondering what her husband was up to now.

"Naw, we just met in the men's room," J.T. said with a laugh. "Roger's a chaplain, and we got to talking . . . about Chad."

Her arms were still folded, and she kept looking at her husband.

"I was telling Roger I—er—we, could both use someone to talk to."

"Oh."

"So what do you say?"

She shrugged. "I don't know if I'll say something, but that's fine."

Jamison led them to his office, where they sat on a couch while he pulled up a chair. He began, "Why don't you tell me what you're feeling?"

"Well, I'm angry," Marie-Paule answered.

"Why?"

"Because I can't figure out why this is happening to us. When I pray, I don't even know what to tell God for letting this happen."

Jamison nodded. "I understand. Think of it this way. When we say the 'Our Father,' and 'give us this day our daily bread,' we're not just asking for sustenance. We're asking for the strength to face what is challenging us."

She didn't reply.

"So when you pray, imagine you're sitting beside God, watching what he's doing, not sitting across from him opposed to what he's doing, because He is the ultimate healer and Creator."

J.T.'s eyes filled with tears. "I'll be honest with you, Roger. I feel like my faith is shot, because here I am crying, and I shouldn't be. . . Is that a lack of faith?"

"Jesus and Mary cried, too, and it didn't weaken their faith." Jamison continued. "Think about passages from Scripture, where Jesus himself doubts his faith. Can you picture him in the Garden of Gethsemane? He knows what God has in store for him—humiliation, torture and death on the cross, and weeps openly while asking if he can avoid 'drinking from this cup.'"

J.T. gripped his wife's hand while he regained his composure. Finally, he said, "Do a lot of people like us come here and pour out their souls to you?"

"Not really." He smiled. "But you're welcome anytime you feel the need."

"Thanks." They shook hands and left him.

In the hall, J.T. said to his wife, "I don't know about you, but I got more spirituality out of meeting him than from a lifetime of going to church."

"Good."

On the Wednesday following surgery, a neurosurgeon began removing the catheters draining Chad's head, at the same time monitoring him closely to see if pressure was remaining normal in his skull. By Thursday morning, they also pulled his ventilator tube, allowing him to breathe on his own.

And just like that, he woke up.

Marie-Paule was sitting next to him. She heard him say, "J'ai froid." She turned to the nearby nurse.

"He's cold."

"Oh, it sounds like he's just mumbling."

"No, he told me he's cold. He's speaking French."

"Are you telling me your son speaks *French*? How am I going to communicate with him?" the nurse said, genuinely concerned.

"It's okay. I grew up in Belgium. Chad's bi-lingual . . . Hopefully he'll remember his English, too."

Marie-Paule couldn't believe two words could fill her with such joy. She wasn't sure herself if Chad could still speak English as well. In fact, when she broke the news to J.T., she said, "If Chad can't speak English any more, you may have to finally learn good French."

By that afternoon, however, Chad did have a message— in English—for his dad. "Thanks for not letting me die."

He also began chatting with his doctors and nurses, who were eager to evaluate his mental faculties. He was asked if he knew what had happened to him and where he was. "Yes, I had a bad headache, and was put in an ambulance. But I'm not sure what happened after that. And now I'm in Latrobe Hospital."

"No," his mother said. "You're in Children's Hospital in Pittsburgh."

"Oh . . . Now it all makes sense."

"What does?"

"All the nurses and doctors have Pittsburgh on their I.D.'s. I kept wondering why they'd do that if we were in Latrobe."

"We've been here for the better part of a week, honey.

The doctors did surgery on your head, and now, well, they're learning how well you did."

He also noticed his younger sister for the first time. "Hey Sasha."

She walked shyly up to his bed. "Hi. How do you feel?"

"Mostly tired."

"Uh huh."

"What's new with you?"

"Well, I was just wondering what you want for your birthday."

"My birthday's not for two more months, Sasha."

"I know. But tell me anyway."

"What I want is too expensive for you; you wouldn't be able to afford it."

"Tell me anyway."

"Okay, an iPod."

"Here you go."

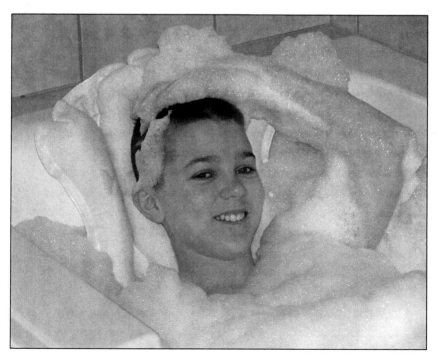

Post surgery, sudsed up in the tub.

Chad's eyes lit up as he opened the package. "But how am I going to listen? I can't put the ear plugs in with my head all bandaged up."

"We can just play it without earplugs," she said.

"Is there already music on it?"

"Yeah," she giggled. "I downloaded some soft stuff at Uncle Blake's."

"Cool." She showed him how to begin the songs.

"So you're really feeling okay?" Sasha again asked.

"Yeah, except for one thing. Mom, can somebody take these diapers off? I feel silly wearing them."

His parents arranged for a potty-seat to be delivered. They lowered Chad from his bed and led him to the seat. But he couldn't pee.

They helped him back into bed, and handed him a urine bottle. They even drew the curtains to give him more privacy. No luck.

Finally, the nurse said, "We have to give him a catheter. He has to pass his urine."

When they inserted the first tube, Chad howled in protest. Worse, he still couldn't relieve himself. The nurse was trying a second, thinner, tube when Chad said, "If you don't stop it, I'm going to *slap* you!"

"I know it hurts, honey, but we have to do it," the nurse replied. Her name was Corinne.

The catheter eventually worked, but Chad detested it more than the diapers.

A speech therapist then came by to gauge whether Chad's swallowing reflex would allow him to begin eating food again. He had no trouble swallowing liquids and soft foods, and eventually was given a Popsicle.

It quickly became obvious, however, that he hadn't gone through the delicate surgery unscathed. Because the tumor and operation involved the right side of his brain, the left side of his body reflected the side effects. Initially, he was weak as an infant, particularly his left arm. Moreover, when a doctor would lift it and ask "Whose hand?", Chad would say "It's yours."

The physician reminded the Scanlons such short-circuits were to be expected following brain surgery, and that most would diminish or disappear altogether once Chad underwent physical therapy.

Their son also was under the influence of powerful medications, and was having trouble shaking off their side effects. For instance, he was prone to repeating himself and his short-term memory was marginal.

But by Friday morning, almost a week after his surgery, Chad was moved out of ICU to continue recovering on the 10th Floor. When the catheter was finally removed, Marie-Paule said, "I'll bet you're happy that's out. That poor nurse who you yelled at for putting it in, she's probably still sad from you scolding her."

"What nurse, mom? I don't remember yelling at any nurse . . . What did I say?"

"You told her to stop, or you'd *slap* her."

His face reddened. "I need to see her," Chad said. "You need to find Corrine. I need to apologize."

J.T. said he'd go back down to ICU to look for her. When he found Corrine, he said, "Chad really feels bad about what he said to you the other day. He wants you to come up so he can apologize."

"He doesn't have to do that," she said. "I'm sure it was just his medication."

"Even so, he'd like to see you."

She stared at J.T. "Okay. I'll come up on my break."

When she did, Chad said, "I'm sorry for being mean to you. My mom says I threatened to slap you for putting in the catheter. I would never do something like that."

"I know you wouldn't, Chad. Patients sometimes say the darnedest thing when they're hurting."

By the one-week anniversary of his surgery, Chad was encouraged to slide out of bed and go for a walk. The incen-

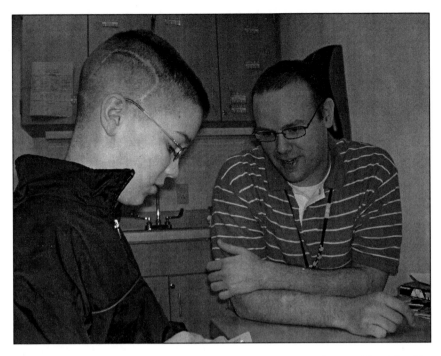

During surgery, Chad's optic nerve was affected, leaving him blind in the left half of both eyes. Here he is undergoing therapy at The Children's Institute in Pittsburgh.

tive was a visiting miniature pony, one of several animals brought in to Children's periodically to raise patients' spirits. Chad thought the whole notion silly. Nevertheless, he used the occasion to walk one hundred feet with an assist from J.T. and Marie-Paule.

The medical staff was amazed by the speed of his recovery, which his parents attributed to their son's fitness from jumping rope. There was no sign of swelling in his brain; in fact, no major complications at all. What did become obvious, however, was Chad's ongoing difficulty with the left side of his body. Whenever his parents walked with him down a hallway, he tended to drift to his left, even turning into rooms other than his own. They would later learn the tumor and subsequent bleeding had affected his peripheral vision to the point he couldn't see objects to his left in either eye. An ophthalmologist would eventually tell the family, "It's not that he sees black in the left half of both eyes; he doesn't see anything. We call that field-cut vision. But with training, he'll learn to compensate."

The Scanlons were determined to learn more about Chad's cancer. They began by enlisting the help of several family members and friends. "Find out all you can about this disease," they wrote in an email, "so we know if Dr. Hemminger and Children's are Chad's best hope." Their request came after Dr. Hemminger, this time with Perry at her side, again met with the Scanlons in private to discuss Chad's treatment. She told them she and her colleagues believed Chad had a malignant tumor called a PNET (Primitive Neuroectodermal Tumor), and the survival rate was 33 percent. "If that's the case, we're going to have to radiate the spine, the head, the whole nervous system," she said.

J.T. had heard enough. "Goddamnit!" He threw his water bottle against the wall behind Hemminger and Perry, bursting it over the floor. He stormed out of the room.

On Friday, after Chad had been moved to the 10th floor, Dr. Hemminger again convened a meeting. This time she sat down with Marie-Paule, J.T. and his brothers Blake and Daniel. She told them the tumor diagnosis had evolved, and it was leaning toward a type of brain cancer called "glioblastoma." She recommended Chad undergo targeted radiation on the remaining tumor mass five days a week along with a daily chemo pill for six weeks straight. She didn't anticipate any major side effects from the chemo, but did warn that the recommended dose of radiation could cause cognitive learning disabilities down the road because Chad was so young.

The solitary grain of good news? "The treatment's a lot easier," Dr. Hemminger explained, because it didn't require radiating his entire nervous system. Then the bombshell.

"However, Chad now has only a five percent survival rate."

Marie-Paule was stunned—and uncharacteristically blunt. "I'm sorry, but I hate seeing you. I don't like you, you're always the bearer of bad news."

The other people in the room thought Hemminger took it quite well.

"Look, it's not personal," J.T. explained. "It's just every time you come in you have bad news for us, and we just hate to see you. We just hate when you walk through that door because you don't have anything good to tell us."

They also asked Dr. Hemminger whom she would ask for a second opinion if Chad were her child. She gave them the name of an associate at another hospital, but cautioned that if they sought a hundred opinions, half would come back with the PNET diagnosis and half the glioblastoma. Either way, the grim prognosis wouldn't improve.

Near the end of the meeting, Marie-Paule said, "Okay, we're just going to concentrate on the treatment. And he may be in the five percent. I don't want to hear anything else."

"You're right," Hemminger said. "Focus on that."

Marie-Paule then asked her, "How do you tell a kid he has a *five-percent* chance of surviving this thing? How do you tell him what he's going to have to go through?"

"Well, you have to trust your child. He's stronger than you think."

Afterward, the Scanlons began digesting all the treatment options. The news on glioblastomas accumulated by their "search group" was indeed grim. Although a rare form of cancer—less than two or three cases per 100,000 people— glioblastomas grew as if pumped with steroids. And actual cases of survival were alarmingly few.

There was also the question of picking traditional chemo and radiation treatment over "alternative" medicine. Several members of the Scanlons' extended family had contracted cancer and chosen to simply eat a strict organic diet boosted by "natural" supplements. J.T. and Marie-Paule even debated combining the two approaches: modern medicine accompanied by holistic treatments. However, Dr. Hemminger counseled against giving Chad herbal remedies because there was no clinical research indicating they did any good. "There's also no way of knowing if they'd do harm to Chad," she added.

In the end, the Scanlons decided to go the medically approved route.

They were still agonizing over picking the right time and place to tell Chad about his diagnosis. As it turned out, the decision was made for them. On the following Monday, less than two weeks following his surgery, Chad was preparing to be transferred to the nearby Children's Institute in Squirrel Hill to begin rehabilitation. Marie-Paule had spent the night with him, and was talking to J.T. on her cell phone to plan when they would meet that morning. Meanwhile, she could overhear an aide who'd come in to bathe Chad casually mentioning "chemo and radiation."

Marie-Paule caught the woman's attention and stared. The aide left without saying another word.

Chad quickly turned to her. "Mom, do I have cancer?"

"J.T., I have to go. Chad has questions."

She looked directly into her son's eyes. "Well, Chad, the cause of your headaches is the tumor that you had in your brain, and the tumor is cancer and it eventually bled, and that's why you had to be rushed to the hospital and have emergency surgery. Now they removed what they could, but there could be some left because it was really hard to see because it's deep in your brain and there was a lot of blood. But, yes, you do have cancer."

She saw fear sweep over his face, so she quickly continued. "Chad, we already have a plan of attack. There is treatment we can try. There is going to be radiation and chemo but the doctor told us the chemo will be easy. It's a pill, and there is medication you can take so it doesn't make you sick.

As for radiation, I'm not sure how you're going to do that or what's going to happen with that, but you're going to have radiation. Maybe we need to talk to the doctor to explain what exactly is going to happen during that treatment."

For the first time, tears streamed down Chad's cheeks. "Mom, I remember a catechism teacher told us she had cancer and had radiation, and it was terrible because her skin was burnt, and it was so sore and she was all red and it really burned. I don't want to get burned."

"Well, maybe we need to talk to the doctors about that and see what they have to say."

He appeared to be deep in thought for nearly a minute.

"You know what, Mom? In religion class, Mr. Lawson told us that Pope John Paul, when he learned about his disease, and he was really sick, said that he will be okay because he will never suffer like Jesus did . . . And that's the same for me. I'm not going to suffer like Jesus, or Grandma. I'll be fine."

(A few years earlier, Chad's grandmother, Ellen, with whom he had a special bond, had contracted Lou Gehrig's Disease, or ALS. It had killed her in little over a year.)

Later that morning, the social worker happened to come by. Marie-Paule said to him, "Perry, Chad knows now what is going on with his situation and he has questions, and I'm not sure if we can find Dr. Hemminger or somebody to answer them."

"Well, just ask me and maybe I can answer it."

Chad expressed his fears about radiation.

"A long time ago the radiation machine they used did burn you," Perry explained. "But now they have the best technology. Here they have one of the newest machines. They'll also give you gel to protect your skin, and you won't get burned."

Chad appeared to be comforted by the explanation, and wiped away his tears. It was the last time he would cry for the foreseeable future.

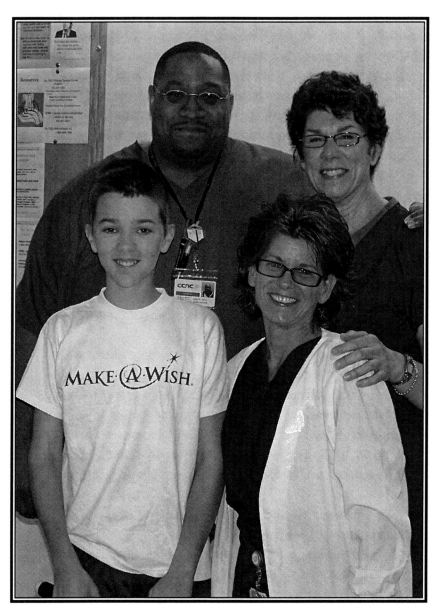

Chad poses with radiation technicians at UPMC.

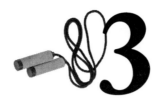

The Children's Institute: A Happy Place

T he Children's Institute in Pittsburgh is a renowned pediatric care center. It was founded under a different name in 1902 to care for a single young boy whose legs had been severed in a train accident. As its outreach grew, it treated children for polio—the scourge of the mid 1900s—and even adults for periods of time. However, in 1998, the center was renamed The Children's Institute to reflect its renewed focus on children facing assorted disabilities. Many, like Chad, undergo rehabilitation until they're healthy enough to be discharged. Others are so severely disabled they essentially become full-time residents.

Chad's goal at The Children's Institute was straightforward: regain strength, stamina and motor skills so he could face head on the adversity of radiation and chemotherapy. At this point, however, Marie-Paule's spirits were sagging, and she was secretly yearning to grab her son and whisk him away to the reassuring confines of their mountain home. Instead, once Chad was transferred to the Institute, they sat side by side on his bed—basically waiting for someone to tell them what they had to do next.

A woman poked her head into their room. "Hi, I'm Meredith. I'll be Chad's case manager."

Marie-Paule smiled despite herself. "Look Chad, someone

who's cheery for once."

"I think you'll find this is a pretty happy place, Mrs. Scanlon, despite the challenges facing some of our patients."

She focused on Chad. "So I understand you're here for physical, speech and occupational therapy, Chad."

"Uh huh."

"I see from your chart that you're going to be undergoing radiation and chemo at some point—"

He nodded.

"And your doctors want you to regain some lost weight, rebuild your muscle tone, and meanwhile give that surgical scar time to heal. Sound about right?"

"I guess so."

"It also says here you may have lost some vision in the left field of both eyes."

"Yeah, I have trouble seeing things to my left."

"Well, don't worry, Chad. That's what the occupational therapy is for. We'll teach you how to compensate for what you can't see by turning your head more as you navigate."

Meredith said to Marie-Paule, "Any other problems I may not be aware of?"

"Well, he's still having some trouble with weakness on his left side. And sometimes he can't tell that his left hand is really his left hand."

Meredith smiled.

"And there are words, or objects I should say, that he now has trouble remembering."

"Give me an example."

"Well, he can remember all sorts of things from before the surgery—friends, relatives, things we've done as a family. . . But he has trouble remembering words he needs to express himself. Like my husband J.T. might ask Chad what a table is, and he won't know."

"I understand, Mrs. Scanlon."

"Please. Call me Marie-Paule."

"Of course. Marie-Paule, again, that's where speech ther-

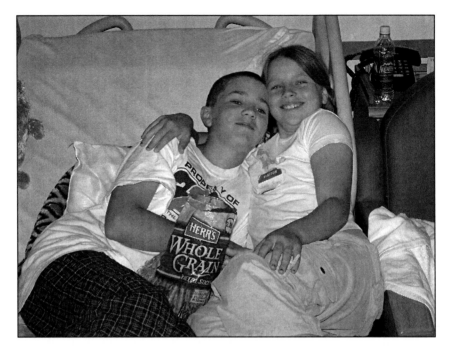

Cuddling with sister Sasha at The Childrens Institute, Pittsburgh.

apy comes in. The therapist will help Chad identify objects by breaking them down into components. So that table you mentioned might first be 'brown,' then 'wood,' then finally 'something we eat on.' And I'm confident that'll help Chad recognize it then as a table."

Marie-Paule could suddenly feel her spirits lifting. *Maybe this isn't another sad place after all.*

Meredith said, "Okay, I think we've covered enough to get started. Are you ready to start work later today, Chad?"

He smiled weakly.

"Good."

As Meredith turned to leave, Marie-Paule walked with her to the hallway. Outside, she said softly, "He may not look it now, but two weeks ago Chad was a very healthy, strong boy, and extremely bright—"

"What's worrying you, Marie-Paule?"

"I'm just wondering if he'll ever be the same. He still gets confused easily, and his strength seems to have disappeared."

Meredith nodded, and put a hand on her shoulder. "I think you'll be surprised how quickly much of the Chad you knew comes back. I'm not worried about his physical strength returning at all—"

"Yes, but will he still be able to learn?"

"Well, time will tell. And I imagine the doctors warned you that radiation at Chad's age could affect his cognitive abilities down the road."

Marie-Paule nodded.

"Why don't we just see how he responds to therapy? I've seen some amazing recoveries in my time here."

"This is a good place?"

"A very good place."

"Thank you. I'm feeling a little more hopeful already."

"You're welcome. Now later on today, Chad will meet his new physical therapist. Her name's Mandy. She'll discuss her plans to make him stronger."

"Okay. Thanks again."

Through physical therapy, Chad needed only several days at The Children's Institute to regain much of his lost strength and agility. On the third day, Mandy asked, "Okay, Chad, what's your next goal?"

"I want to be able to jump rope again."

"Well, okay. I suppose we'll need to get a rope some day and do a couple jumps and see what happens."

"I already have my rope. My Dad brought it from home."

"Oh . . . Well, how about we start with just a couple jumps then, and see how you do?"

His mother handed Chad his jump rope. He began twirling it slowly at first, completing simple two-footed jumps one at a time. Without saying a word, however, he suddenly began doing more complex maneuvers: double-unders—where the rope passes twice under his feet each jump, and crossovers—where his arms form an X with the rope and then separate again on each pass.

"Oh, my God!" Mandy said. "Just a couple jumps, Chad." Everyone in the room was smiling now, none more proudly than Marie-Paule.

Chad's jump-rope skills became such a hit everyone in the Institute wanted to see him perform. So it was quickly incorporated into his daily therapy. And before long, he could manage 240 revolutions per minute in speed skills, not far off from his previous best of 298 rpm. "It's kind of amazing considering what he's gone through, but his mind hasn't forgotten how to do all those jumps, just like he's never forgotten how to tie his own shoe," J.T. told Mandy.

In occupational therapy, Chad was often asked to assemble jigsaw puzzles, a task he once enjoyed without thinking hard. Now, however, he'd go so far with the puzzle and think he was done, when in reality he couldn't actually see some missing pieces. J.T. had to force himself not to help his son.

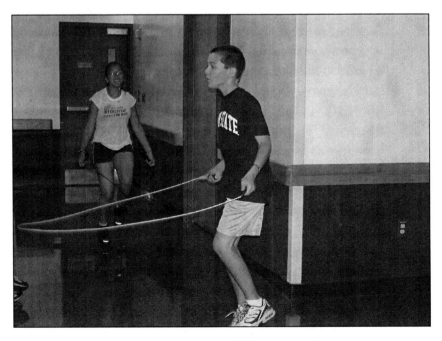

Jumping rope after surgery at The Children's Institute.

Chad thoroughly enjoyed speech therapy, especially when it was tied into card games that he would play with Sasha or his cousins. On the other hand, he never saw the point in one-on-one meetings with a staff psychologist, who asked him questions such as: "Can a cat jump over the moon?" He would tell his mother, "I wanted to tell him 'yes,' just to see the expression on his face."

Nevertheless, after early evaluations of Chad by Institute staff, Marie-Paule and J.T. were amused to hear their son referred to as "a genius." In fact, they were asked to bring him back for re-testing six months after his discharge so evaluators could determine whether Chad's intelligence was still at such a high level. He, himself, was nonchalant about all the attention paid to his mental abilities. "So I answered a few questions right. That doesn't make me a genius."

Chad would eventually befriend a young African-American boy named Peter, who sat next to him in the cafeteria during meals. He was wheel chair bound, and couldn't speak. He also had no visitors, Marie-Paule recalls, so the Scanlons made it their mission to brighten his day whenever and however possible. "One way or another we tried to bring a smile to his face every day," she says.

Normally, though, Chad preferred to take the majority of his meals in his room, surrounded by the never-ending stream of visiting family and friends. Most meals were brought in by those guests. Meanwhile, back on Chestnut Ridge, people had begun swamping the Scanlon house with fresh and frozen dinners. Their refrigerator and freezer were packed with enough meals to last weeks. Their fellow parishioners at St. Boniface had also collected several thousand dollars in donations to help defray the family's expenses. But perhaps most heartening were the legions of faithful who now included Chad on their prayer lists.

Amidst all the outpouring of support, Chad continued to improve. He was particularly pleased the night he received permission to go swimming. It had been an entire week in the making until his scar had finally healed sufficiently. "I just want to go under," he told his mother. "I just want to go under so I can swim like a fish again."

There were other memorable days, sometimes eerily so. One afternoon while at the Institute, Chad needed to have an MRI. Because Children's Hospital was booked, however, the Scanlons were instead directed to nearby Magee Women's Hospital. While Marie-Paule and Chad waited for the procedure, J.T. joined his brothers Blake and Mike for a quick snack in the cafeteria.

During lunch, Blake said, "Jimmy, didn't you go to school with that guy over there?"

J.T. turned and saw a former high school classmate, Rick Gnagy. When he walked by, J.T. stood and re-introduced himself.

"What are you doing here, Jimmy?" Gnagy got around to asking.

"Well, my son's getting an MRI. A couple weeks back, Chad was lifeflighted from Latrobe to Children's, where he was diagnosed with a brain tumor. Our doctor, Rachael Hemminger, told us the cancer's called glioblastoma. Although we're at The Children's Institute right now for rehab, the doctors sent us down here today for the MRI. They said they need to see what's going on in his head."

"Man, I'm just the guy you need to talk to," Gnagy said. "My son, Joshua, had brain and spinal cancer. In fact, Hemminger was his doctor. He was just a baby, and they gave him zero chance of survival."

"What happened?"

"It was basically a miracle, because he was too young for radiation, and was even given the wrong chemotherapy for his type of cancer. Just the same, he's cured."

"That's incredible, Rick."

"Yep."

"So what are you doing at Magee?"

"I work here . . . In fact, I'd say it's more than chance that brought you here today, Jimmy. We both have sons treated by the same doctor. I'd say we were meant to meet today. Come to think of it, why don't you and your wife come over to the house some evening and meet my wife Ashley? When you do, I'll show you the videotape made of Joshua when he was on The 700 Club."

"Oh yeah?"

"Yeah. On the show they called him "The Miracle Baby.""

The men exchanged contact information, shook hands and parted ways.

Shortly thereafter, Ashley Gnagy called Marie-Paule at The Children's Institute, told her who she was and why she was calling. "Marie-Paule, now I know you don't know me, but I need to tell you something amazing. While your husband was bumping into Rick at Magee, I was in Monroeville giving a talk about my experience with my son, which was a truly miraculous healing. When Joshua was sick, Rick and I both had a vision of an angel who said, 'Joshua will be fine.' And eventually he was, even though he was given no chance of reaching his first birthday. Anyway, during my talk in Monroeville, a woman in the audience asked me if we could stop and pray for a little boy she knew who also had brain cancer. So I asked her his name . . . "

"And—"

"She said 'Chad.'"

The story had a powerful effect on Marie-Paule. *How weird that someone we didn't know asked Ashley to pray for Chad at the same time J.T. was meeting up with Rick. Maybe this means we're going to have a miracle, too. Otherwise, why would we be meeting these people?*

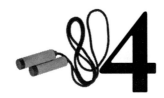

The Wedding

From the first day in The Children's Institute, Marie-Paule had one question she would ask the administrative staff every chance she had: "We have a special wedding coming up. Do you think we can get permission to attend it with Chad?"

At least initially, no one was willing to commit. But neither did they rule out the possibility. So each afternoon, Marie-Paule would again ask, "Do you think we'll be able to go to this special wedding?"

An administrator told her, "I don't see why not, but we'll see."

The wedding was special because it was between family friend Aurora Valdez and Kevin McCormick, J.T.'s cousin. Marie-Paule had planned the bridal shower for Aurora the night in July when Chad had first gotten ill. Since they hadn't been able to celebrate at the shower, at least they hoped they could attend the wedding.

Aurora's employer, Muriel Costello, was determined that the Scanlons join in the festivities, which would be hosted under tents at her Ligonier home. In fact, she had basically adopted the Scanlons after learning of Chad's cancer. Over the phone, she told Marie-Paule, "I am so upset about Chad being sick. If you ever need me, I'm a good grandma. I can

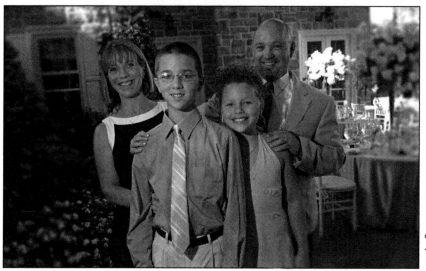

Jeff Swensen Photographer

The Scanlon family enjoys a special time at the wedding.

spend a night. Whatever you need, let me know."

"Thank you, Mrs. Costello. They tell us, if everything's all right, we might be able to come to the wedding."

"Wonderful. Now you tell those people at the Institute I'll take care of everything the afternoon of the wedding."

Marie-Paule laughed. "Everything?"

"*Everything.*" And then they finalized the particulars over the phone.

Thanks to Chad's rapid progress in rehab, he was granted approval to attend the wedding with his parents. Marie-Paule told Chad the day before his Uncle Blake would be driving into Pittsburgh to pick them all up for the ride to his house, where they would get Sasha and then proceed to Ligonier. So as Chad underwent therapy the following morning, he couldn't help picturing how much fun they'd have in a few hours.

By noon, therapy was over, and Marie-Paule and J.T. waited anxiously with Chad for their ride.

At the appointed time, they left The Children's Institute and walked outside. A stretch limousine was parked in front.

The driver stepped out and walked up to them. He said to their son, "Are you Chad Scanlon?'

"Yes."

"Well, young man, I'm going to be your driver for the day."

"You don't look like Uncle Blake."

He laughed. "I understand, sir. But nevertheless, I and this limousine are at your disposal for the rest of the evening, courtesy of Mrs. Costello."

"Wow. You're coming with us to the wedding?"

"And bringing you home afterward, Chad."

The family piled into the limousine. An hour later, when it pulled into the real Uncle Blake's driveway, Chad and Marie-Paule opened the sunroof and stood up to wave to Sasha, who was waiting at the house. She was as excited as Chad about the wedding, if not more so. The minute she stepped into the car, she began rolling on the seat and pushing buttons, saying, "This is awesome."

The family was driven to their home, where they showered and dressed. Chad wore a suit, and Sasha the dress she'd worn the night of Aurora's shower. When they were ready,

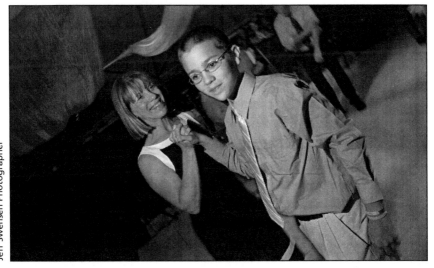

Jeff Swensen Photographer

Chad and Marie-Paule hit the dance floor.

the driver proceeded to the Costello home. Although Aurora and Kevin were the official guests of honor, because of Chad's condition, he may have been more of a star than they. The band had been briefed in advance and made sure to play all of his favorite ABBA songs, and it seemed that every young lady in attendance requested a dance with him. Asked about the wedding the next day, J.T. told a friend: "We all had a great time. We forgot everything. We were a normal family again last night."

In fact, they overstayed their Cinderella outing. Instead of returning to the Institute by the eleven p.m. curfew, they didn't come back until 12:30 a.m. Officials at the Institute overlooked the minor infraction, however, especially when the Scanlons retrieved armfuls of floral arrangements from the limousine. Mrs. Costello insisted they take and distribute the wedding flowers to the other children, who enjoyed the elaborate bouquets the entire following week.

With the wedding behind him, Chad had recuperated enough to begin the daunting series of radiation treatments he was scheduled to have. At 10 a.m. each day, he would shuttle over to UPMC Hospital to have his head radiated, and then return for therapy in the afternoon. The radiation was targeted in a circular one-inch band running from ear to ear. Although he wasn't expected to lose hair from his oral chemotherapy, the radiation was expected to affect him. And it eventually did, causing his hair to fall out with edges so defined Chad looked as if he'd received a precision horizontal buzz cut.

Fatigue was another side effect, which made his afternoon physical and occupational therapy a challenge at times. But he endured the regimen without complaint, and after nearly a month at The Children's Institute, he was finally ready to be discharged. The downside was that he would have to be driven back during morning rush hour five days a week and undergo therapy three of those afternoons.

Moreover, the day of his discharge began ominously. He complained to his parents of a headache, and pressure behind his eyes. When they called Dr. Hemminger, she told them Chad would need an emergency MRI just to be safe. But once again, Children's Hospital had no openings. So Marie-Paule and J.T. took Chad to Magee Hospital. By this time, Chad was understandably apprehensive. "Mom, is the tumor causing my headache?"

"That's what we're going to find out today, sweetie."

He had begun to dread MRI's because he was forced to lie headfirst in the tight confines of the machine for up to three hours.

Fortunately, the Scanlons were met at Magee by a trio of sympathetic nurses: Darcy, Emily and JoEllen. Darcy prepped Chad for the test, but because it was late in the afternoon and her shift over, she apologized and said she would have to leave. JoEllen took over the procedure and completed it.

When the long test was done, Marie-Paule and J.T. were surprised to find Darcy in the visitors' lounge after all. "I thought you were done hours ago," J.T. teased.

"I was. But I couldn't go home. I just needed to know that he'd gotten through and was okay." She added, "How did it go?"

J.T. shrugged. "We're still waiting to hear from Dr. Hemminger."

And then her call came. "I've reviewed the scans. I don't think there's any problem. Go home."

Instead, the Scanlons first returned to The Children's Institute, where Chad's fellow jump-ropers from Holy Trinity were scheduled to perform an exhibition. Because he was in no shape to jump with them, he remained on the sidelines and cheered with the other Institute patients in the audience. It wasn't the way he hoped to finish his last day as a resident, but he went home with a smile on his face nonetheless.

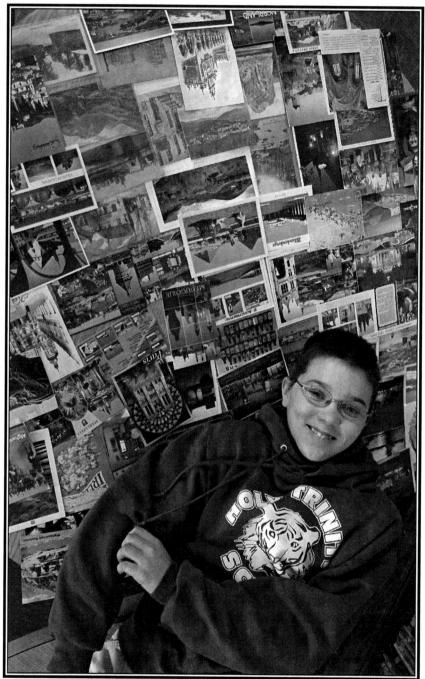

Chad was so fascinated with geography he eventually accumulated postcards from all 50 states and 79 different countries.

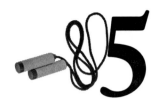

Peaks and Valleys

Chad came home to Chestnut Ridge on August 18, slightly over a month following his surgery. Ahead of him was another month of radiation—five days a week—along with a daily chemo pill. It soon became obvious his appetite was being dampened by the treatments.

At a picnic hosted by his jump-rope coach, he couldn't force himself to eat. And later that week, when his mother made chicken Alfredo, his favorite, he still couldn't stomach the idea of eating. "Nothing tastes good anymore," he explained. Well, maybe chocolate. Even so, Chad began to lose weight, which he couldn't afford to do.

To remedy the situation, Dr. Hemminger prescribed an appetite "booster." She told Marie-Paule, "Chad has a choice of this medicine; he can take 10 pills a day, or a couple drops in a glass of water." Much to her chagrin, Chad opted for the capsules. "I'll take the ten pills. At least they don't taste bad like the liquid medicine."

Afterward, his appetite swelled to the point his parents actually worried he was eating too much. But at least he was eating again.

By now, J.T. had returned to his lineman's job. So initially, Marie-Paule relied on friends and family to drive her to Pittsburgh each day until she became comfortable making the trip on her own.

I rode passenger with her early on while she drove, partly to show her a few shortcuts along the way. That day at Children's, Chad underwent radiation without a hitch and then came outside to the visitors' lounge. Waiting for him was his radiation oncologist. "I hear you're pretty good at jumping rope. Care to show me a few moves?"

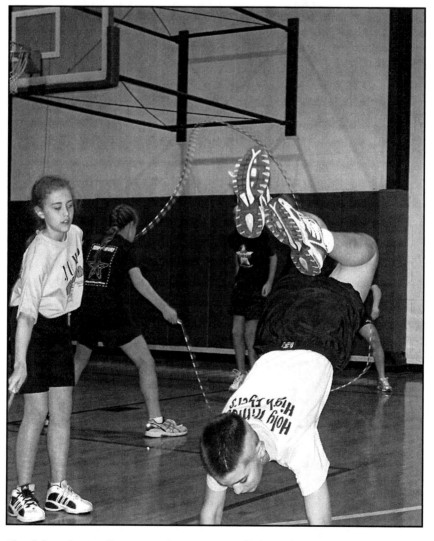

Chad hand-standing at a jump rope clinic a few months after his surgery.

"Sure."

Chad stepped out into the hall, took his rope and, without a bit of self-consciousness, began going through his routine for several minutes. The doctor shook his head in wonderment. "Good grief, Chad. I had no idea. You *are* a phenom."

He smiled shyly.

This was a good day.

But over time, the strain of the commute and his treatment began to wear on Chad. One day, on the way in, he balked completely. "I don't want to do radiation any more," he told his mother.

"Why?"

"Lying there reminds me of being in the MRI. It's scary."

Marie-Paule nodded. "I know, Chad, but I don't think the doctors are going to be too happy about you skipping radiation."

When they arrived at radiology later that morning, Chad's fears boiled to the surface. Nurses came out to inform Marie-Paule after only a few minutes. "What's wrong?" she asked.

"Chad probably had a small panic attack in the radiology lab," the nurse said. "He said he couldn't breathe. He was having a pretty bad time."

"So what are we going to do?"

"Well, the radiologist said he could skip today, but he'll still have to come back tomorrow as scheduled."

Marie-Paule thought a moment. "And if it happens again tomorrow?"

"You should probably talk to him when you get home; find out what he's afraid of."

So that evening, after Marie-Paule told J.T., he talked briefly with his son. The next day he called off work and went to radiation with them both. At UPMC, J.T. walked with Chad into the radiology lab and held his hand before the treatment. His son was clearly nervous. "Look, buddy, what's going on? You've been doing this radiation for a while. What's bothering you?"

"I don't know. I just don't want to do it. I'm tired of it . . . I'm done."

J.T. smiled, but without blinking an eye said, "Well, you're not done, buddy. You've got to finish this, see it the whole way through."

Chad reluctantly agreed to try, so J.T. left. However, he still couldn't force himself to lie passively through the treatment, and the session threatened to conclude as badly as the day before. His father again came into the room and tried a different tact. "Look, pal, remember what we talked about last night? We made a deal. I told you if you kept up with radiation, I'd stop chewing tobacco. So if you aren't going to keep your end of the deal today, I'm going down to the store to buy a can of snuff."

Chad let his Dad's ultimatum sink in. Then he underwent the radiation. In fact, he would do so without protest from then on.

MRI's were another story, though. Chad had grown so anxious over his latest one it had to be cancelled. Dr. Hemminger suggested giving him Valium, a mild sedative, before the next attempt, and Marie-Paule agreed to give him a pill before leaving home. Instead of calming him, however, the sedative appeared to have the opposite effect. Chad giggled, said he had to use the restroom every five minutes, and basically refused to lie still.

A day later, the doctors gave Chad a short-term sedative when he arrived for the test. This time he woke up part way through the MRI. They gave him a second dose. Before the test was completed, he woke up a second time, and the MRI had to be called off.

On his third attempt in a week, doctors decided they had no choice but to give Chad general anesthesia to put him in a deep sleep. While he and his mother waited for the procedure in the lounge, a woman came up to Marie-Paule and handed her a medal of an angel. Thinking the woman must be selling the medal, Marie-Paule interrupted a cell phone call to her sister by saying, "No, thank you," and handed it back.

The woman replied, "No, it's for you." Then she turned and left.

Several minutes later, the woman returned, this time with her mother. "Hi, my name's Samantha."

"Oh, you're the one who gave me the medal. Why did you do that? Do I look that desperate that you thought I needed an angel?"

"No. But when you were on the phone, God told me to give you my angel. When I was a little girl, I was born with a congenital brain condition. I wasn't supposed to live. But here I am. And God told me to give you my angel because you need hope and strength."

Marie-Paule couldn't help laughing, "Wow, God talked to you about me. Great!"

It wasn't the last time people of faith would walk up to her and hand over medals, explaining how they had survived life-threatening illnesses. She thought, *Why would all these people be giving me these medals if Chad wasn't meant to be all right, too?*

Afterward, Chad was given anesthesia and finally completed the MRI. The very next day, he went back to school for his afternoon classes. It was early September, and he had already missed the first week. News came while he and classmates were exercising on the school playground. His mother received a call on her cell phone. Afterward, she said, "Chad, the nurse called about your MRI."

"And?"

"She said there was lots of scar tissue—but no spreading."

He hugged her tightly, and instantly there were high-fives all around the playground.

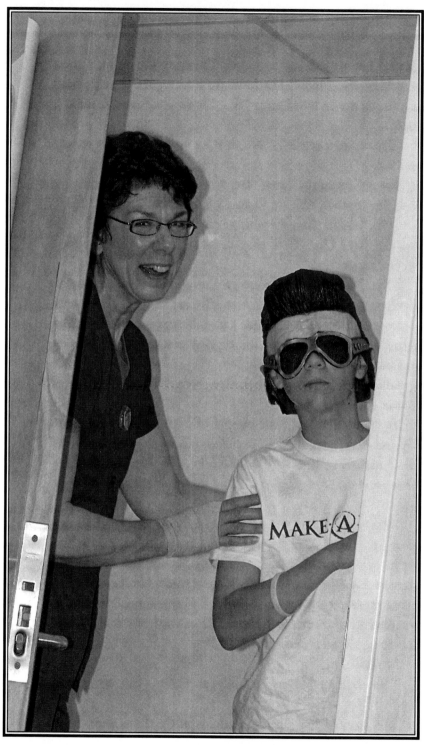

Chad wearing gag Elvis mask on radiology visit after his hair fell out, fall 2006.

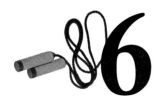

The New Normal

Chad's greatest joy came from returning to school, even if it was only weekday afternoons due to his continuing trips to Pittsburgh for radiation and periodic rehab. By the end of September, however, the radiation was temporarily over and he had a month reprieve from chemotherapy. October was a pleasant distraction all the way until Halloween, when Chad restarted chemo, this time at an even higher dose. As usual, he went to The Children's Institute for rehab that morning, then to school in the afternoon. Everyone was anticipating the Halloween Party following classes, but his stomach began hurting and he was forced to go home. Marie-Paule checked with his physician and consequently gave him a boost of anti-nausea medication, which did the trick.

That evening, he joined Sasha and his classmates for a night of Halloweening followed by the Scanlon tradition of going out for Chinese afterwards. The combination of Halloween candy and General Chao's chicken could've upset any child's stomach, but Chad came through with flying colors.

By early November, Chad was taking chemo pills five days in a row, followed by five weeks off. Doctors had also begun monitoring his blood closely, to make sure his platelet, red and white cell counts hovered around normal levels. And just like that, he began losing his hair one day. Not from the chemo, but the aftereffects of radiation. "Chad," his mother said, "it's just coming out in a half-moon pattern on your head. It almost looks like you were wearing a sweat band too tight." She added, "The doctors asked if you'd like a wig."

"No! I don't want anything."

"Okay."

All the same, the next appointment with his radiologist, he wore an Elvis Presley rubber hair-do and sunglasses. His costume brought down the house.

Meanwhile, at Holy Trinity, Principal Margaret Hoffer offered to make an exception in Chad's case to the school's no-hats' rule. He replied, "No, the rule's the rule."

His classmates, however, came up with a novel idea to make Chad feel more at home with his hair loss. Two sixth-grade girls suggested that students at Holy Trinity could shave their heads as a show of unity for Chad and perhaps even raise money for charity in the process. Mrs. Hoffer appreciated the idea of making Chad feel better, but nixed the notion of doing it to raise money. "This way anyone who wants to shave his head can do so without worrying about the money issue," she said.

So, when Chad showed up for class on the afternoon of November 7, the school secretary instead directed his mother and him to the cafeteria. There, he was startled to see twenty-four individuals—including three girls and two male teachers—having their heads shaved. The instant the assembled students and teachers saw him, they stood and cheered.

He whispered to his mother, "It's really not necessary."

"I know, Chad. But it probably makes them feel good. Just so you know they're thinking of you, that you're not alone in this."

"Oh. That's nice."

One young first-grader was inspired to ask his mother if he could have *his* head shaved.

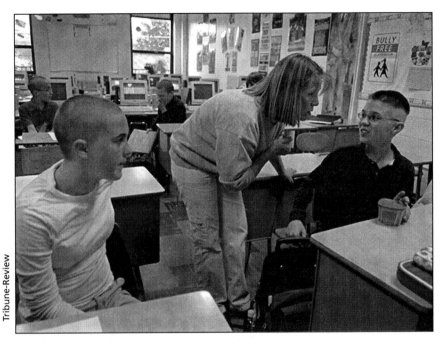

Tribune-Review

Marie-Paule speaks to Chad in his classroom at Holy Trinity Elementary School while a female classmate listens. A number of Chad's classmates cut off their hair and donated it to Locks of Love in Chad's honor, as a way to help him feel more at ease while in school during his second round of chemotherapy, fall 2006.

"Do you really know why you want to do this? You don't have to shave your head?"

"I want to."

"What's the reason?"

"I want to do it for Chad, so he feels good and knows I love him. That's all."

His mother had heard enough. "Then you can do it."

News of the event reached the local newspaper, which sent a reporter to do a follow-up story. The photo featured Chad sitting at a desk next to fellow sixth-grader Elizabeth Bigsby, who had undergone a buzz cut herself. She donated her formerly long brown hair to Locks of Love, which provides hairpieces to underprivileged children who've lost their own hair through illness. "He's one of my best friends,"

Elizabeth explained. "I just thought it was something I should do for him . . . I thought this in a way would make him feel comfortable being with us."

Fellow classmate Terry Norton pooh-poohed his own sacrificial crew cut, saying, "I didn't have much hair to begin with. After I saw Chad like that, I just felt really bad for him, so I thought I'd make him feel better by shaving my head."

This turned out to be just Chapter One in Chad's story as far as the media was concerned. The same newspaper eventually heard of Chad's fascination with geography. As he grew up, he toyed with becoming a marine biologist, cartographer or mapmaker. He had even begun a post card collection from countries of the world before he was sick. Now, he feared he might never travel in person to parts of the globe he'd always wanted to explore. Consequently, his aunt dreamed up the idea of gathering postcards from every state and nation possible. News of her quest swept through his school and across the Internet, and soon postcards from distant lands began pouring into his parents' mailbox. At first, he stored them in a candy box. Then a wooden crate was required.

As 2006 drew to a close, his collection had grown to represent all 50 states and 79 countries. Every continent was represented except Antarctica. U.S. soldiers who had read postings of his growing collection sent cards from Iraq and Afghanistan. He said, "Just seeing how much people care that they would send me things, the soldiers especially . . . That they take the time, with everything they already have on their plate, to add something and send me a card is very meaningful."

His mother said in the article there was plenty of inspiration to go around. "He's teaching me so much by his strength and by his positive attitude. He keeps on going with everything. He never used his condition to say 'poor me,' or 'I don't want to do some work.' He just does it all, and he just says 'I'm fine.' I think he's had a lot to teach us adults."

Over Thanksgiving and Christmas, Chad continued to fare well. His mornings began not with breakfast typically, but downing up to eleven pills: anti-nausea, appetite boosters, chemo, and a mild relaxant. Except for a few minor side effects—including broken leg capillaries from scratching an itch overnight—his health was stable. An MRI in October showed no sign of his tumor spreading, just the usual accumulation of scar tissue.

As December rolled around, Marie-Paule asked Dr. Hemminger if another scan of Chad's brain was due. "No, let's wait until March," she said. "There might still be some swelling from the radiation, which we might confuse with the tumor. I suggest waiting until we're sure everything's settled down in there. Six months after radiation is a good time to check, and that'll be sometime in early March."

Meanwhile, offers to help Chad continued rolling in. One organization, United Bowhunters of Pennsylvania, arranged a free hunting trip for Chad in North Carolina. In fact his whole family was welcome to go along. So on December 6, the Scanlons loaded up their Expedition and drove south to Selma, North Carolina.

Their host was Buck Walthrip, owner of a guide service. He had several other clients visiting that week, but he spent much of his time seeing that Chad's hunt went well. By many measures, it did. He shot a doe his first morning, and a young buck later that afternoon.

But late on the second afternoon, it was a mature buck that had Buck and J.T. excited for Chad. Although the sun had set, and daylight all but disappeared, they urged him to shoot the buck, which was far off and facing away—far from an ideal shot. Buck wasn't worried about Chad wounding the deer, because he could later use his beagle to trail the buck if necessary.

At their urging, Chad studied the buck for a long time. But he declined to shoot. "It's a bad angle," he concluded.

Both men told him to reconsider, so he mounted the rifle

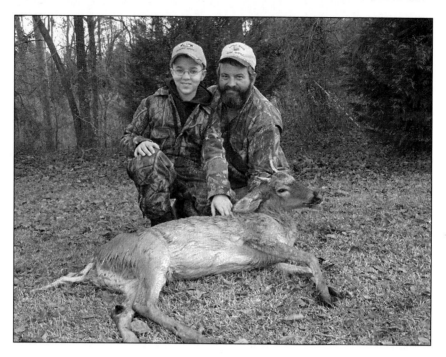

Chad was tickled after shooting this spike buck in North Carolina with his guide and dad in the blind.

a second time. They continued whispering advice, and the seconds ticked by, but he again lowered the gun—without apologizing. "It's still a bad angle. I'm not shooting him."

J.T. was exasperated on the one hand—but not for long. On the ride back to camp, after he had time to think, he told his son, "That was a good decision. Peer pressure doesn't work on you, does it? . . . Way to go, Chad."

Another organization that learned of Chad's condition was the Make-A-Wish Foundation. It has a long history of fulfilling the dreams of seriously ill children. Even so, when Marie-Paule first learned from a Children's Institute employee that Make-A-Wish was interested in helping Chad, she had reservations. "Does this mean you think he's terminal?"

"No," the employee told her. "He's simply eligible for

whatever they can do."

Two volunteers for Make-A-Wish, Tricia and Carolyn, made the initial contact with the Scanlons, and immediately impressed them with their warmth and sincerity.

On their first visit to Chestnut Ridge, the two volunteers asked Chad to draw a picture of what he dreamed of doing. "Well, I'd really like to see more of Europe. I've been to my mom's home in Belgium a few times, but I'd like to see other countries like Italy."

The women looked at each other. Then Tricia said, "I'm sorry, Chad, but Make-A-Wish doesn't offer international trips anymore. There are issues with insurance and medical care for kids like you when you travel out of the country." She continued, "We also can't build you a house, or any other structure, for that matter."

"So I guess air-conditioning at my school is out of the question, then?" he said with a shy smile.

"I'm afraid so . . . But what we can do is help you meet a favorite celebrity, buy a pet, or go somewhere in the United States."

"Hmmm," Chad said. "I think I'm going to have to think more about this." And that was how they left it at the time.

But before Chad left on his hunt in North Carolina, Make-A-Wish asked him to attend Shots for Tots, a fundraiser it sponsored in nearby Greensburg. Each year, current and former members of the Pittsburgh Pirates visited a state prison where they shot baskets with sick children and select inmates. Prisoners at the facility read about Chad in the paper and made sure Make-A-Wish extended him an invitation. The event was the same day the Scanlons were headed to North Carolina.

Inmates made breakfast for all the participants, and then everyone went to the gymnasium to shoot baskets. J.T. and Chad were paired against each other in a shooting contest. But the odds were decidedly in Chad's favor. The muscular inmate feeding balls to the pair leaned over and whispered to

J.T., "You know I can't let you win, right?"

Afterward, Marie-Paule was asked to say a few words. "I just want to thank you guys for requesting Chad. And thank you for your prayers." Without being asked, the inmates then gathered round, held hands, and prayed with the family.

Next up on the agenda was Christmas. It was, in J.T.'s estimation, "overwhelming." The only gifts Chad and Sasha asked for beforehand were a digital camera and bibles. However, presents began pouring in from people at Holy Trinity, other organizations, and friends and family. J.T. said, "We told them to give the gifts to other needy kids, but they said 'no,' we want to do it for Chad. It was unbelievable. Kids would raise money, go shopping, and give us the gifts. There were tons of clothes and toys, and CD's and crafts. Chad and Sasha had more stuff under that Christmas tree than we gave them in their entire lives."

Marie-Paule added, "So we kept reminding Chad and Sasha of the real meaning of Christmas, because 'this isn't going to happen again.' That and people just felt they needed to do something because they were moved by Chad's condition."

Monetary gifts for Chad were piling up, too. But except for buying a few fish for his aquarium, he would've preferred to eventually give it all back. In the meantime, he set it aside for Sasha.

In addition, family came visiting from Belgium. Two of Marie-Paule's friends, Robert and Danielle, brought her mother over for an extended visit. She said, "My mother was so relieved at how well Chad was doing. It was great to have them all here over Christmas. They brought a lot of laughter and joy to the house."

And just like that, the holidays receded. The Scanlons were settling back into some sort of normalcy, so Marie-Paule decided to return to teaching French at Holy Trinity. The family celebrated J.T.'s 40th birthday on January 15. But the focus remained on Chad. He was doing well. No headaches, no symptoms at all.

All the more reason for him to focus on his current goal: an upcoming spelling contest at school. Each evening at home, he would ask his mother to test him with new and more complex words.

There were other diversions as well. Buck Walthrip, their hunting guide from North Carolina, had set up a booth at the Harrisburg Sportsmen's Show, a huge convention in Pennsylvania's state capitol. He invited the Scanlons to attend. There they learned about Hunt of a Lifetime, an organization that provided expense-paid trips for sick children. Through intermediaries, the group let the Scanlons know Chad would be eligible for a hunt as far away as Africa. He told his parents, "That would be great to go to Africa, but I couldn't kill anything there. The animals are too pretty."

He did settle on an elk hunt out West the following fall. Meanwhile, Hunt of a Lifetime raised enough donations at the sporting show to give Chad and his family a free hotel room and dinner while they were in town.

And at some point in the New Year, Chad decided to tell Make-A-Wish that he had settled on visiting Hawaii. Plans were set in motion for a trip that June, when he and Sasha would be out of school.

Next, he went to a jump-rope mini tournament in Ohio—where he performed in speed and power competitions—and came home with ribbons. The other attending teams had cheered him on.

His six-month MRI was scheduled for the following Tuesday. All who knew Chad thought it would be a mere formality. He was doing that well. The scan was taken March 5, and again he had to receive general anesthesia during the procedure. When Chad awoke, his mother and father were hovering over him. Afterward, they went to lunch while the results were studied. Then, they returned to Chad, got him out of bed and dressed, and went into Dr. Hemminger's office. Her assistant began checking Chad's eyesight and balance. J.T. stood off to the side observing—and growing increasingly uneasy. *Something just doesn't feel right.*

Finally, Dr. Hemminger sat down with all three. "I've got some bad news. It's coming back."

Chad's head slumped to his chest.

Worried about what she had to say next, Dr. Hemminger then asked the crestfallen teen to step outside for a few moments. Marie-Paule wanted to protest but bit her lip instead. "The atmosphere was so heavy, it just made me cry," she recalled. "I hated that Chad had to leave the room . . . when what I really wanted to do was hold him . . . and he had to go out and sit with *my* girlfriend, who he barely knew." *Omigod, he just learned the tumor's back, he's going to die, and she's sending him away from us so she can talk to us.*

What's going through his mind there, all alone? He just learned that there's no hope, and he's all alone.

Hemminger resumed the prognosis. "I've consulted with my colleagues before meeting with you, because I frankly didn't want to believe what we're seeing now is the tumor."

"And what did they say?" Marie-Paule asked.

"They said, 'Why are you fighting this? It's obvious.'"

None of the Scanlons said a word on the drive home, until J.T. stopped to pick up a pizza for dinner. While waiting, Marie-Paule turned to Chad in the back seat. "Do you feel like crying?"

"Yeah—"

So she got out and sat in back with him, wrapping Chad in her arms. "Just let it go, honey . . . just let it go." And the tears flowed, for only the second time since he learned he had cancer.

They drove to the home of a family friend who was watching Sasha. The second Barb saw them, she embraced Marie-Paule. "We're just so down," J.T. told her. "We're all down. It's like floating around in a bad dream."

The very next day, one of Chad's eyes had trouble focusing, and his mood slumped. As word of Chad's latest prognosis spread, events were re-shuffled to face the new reality. Make-A-Wish told the Scanlons they could leave for Hawaii within days if they wished, and they made new flight and hotel reservations almost overnight.

A week later, the family was off to fulfill Chad's dream vacation. At first no one was very enthusiastic. But in the following week there would be heartfelt moments, like the day Chad fulfilled a lifelong dream by swimming with dolphins in an ocean inlet. He had once written in a school notebook, "To me, dolphins look so happy and free."

Then there was the helicopter ride over volcanoes arranged by his Uncle Blake. Chad tried valiantly to enjoy each and every opportunity that week, but he often found himself so tired by midday a nap was required. Nevertheless, by week's end, no one really wanted to go home and face what lie ahead.

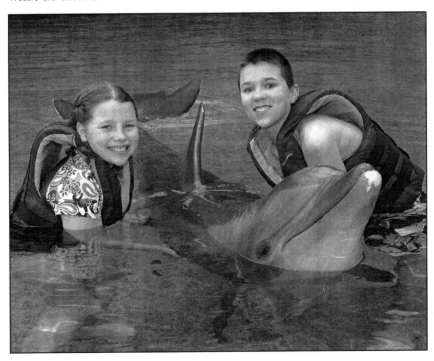

Chad and Sasha swimming with the dolphins in Hawaii.

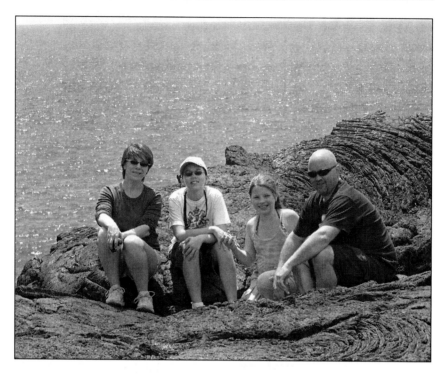

Family photo in Hawaii on lava rock in Volcano National Park.

But they returned as planned to Greater Pittsburgh International Airport, and were met by a strange contingent of well wishers, all of whom had been waiting quite some time due to the flight's delayed arrival. At first, J.T. wasn't even sure who they were. "What the hell's wrong with those people?" he said to his wife. Then he realized the welcoming committee was for his family.

Heading the contingent was Brittany Robinson, an ordained minister and the daughter of J.T.'s supervisor at Allegheny Power. She and her friends were wearing grass skirts, Hawaiian leis, and holding Steeler pom-poms. Brittany told them, "I've been standing here all these hours in a grass skirt, wondering if I'd meet one of my own parishioners. And of course it happened."

An even greater surprise awaited the Scanlons when they pulled down their drive late that evening. First, J.T. noticed his firewood pile had magically grown in his absence. "Look," he said, "someone cut, split and stacked all our logs."

But it was the new three-car garage at the foot of their drive that rendered them speechless. When they'd departed a week ago, all that had stood there was a concrete footer and three-foot block wall J.T. had managed to raise in his spare time. Now the foundation had framed walls, garage door openings, and a brand new shingle roof. "Are we seeing right or what?" he asked Marie-Paule.

A banner hanging from the new structure proclaimed, "Welcome Home!" It was signed by dozens of volunteers who had contributed in one way or another to the garage. The family was greeted by a few family members and friends, who joined them for pizza and beer to talk over their trip. J.T. told one, "You guys certainly put a much-needed smile on our faces. We're happy to be back no matter what."

The garage raising had been spearheaded by two

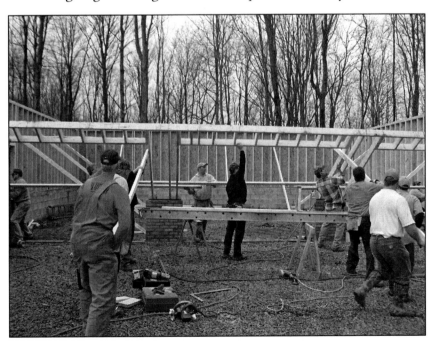

J.T.'s co-workers and friends working on the garage while the family was on Chad's Make-A-Wish trip to Hawaii.

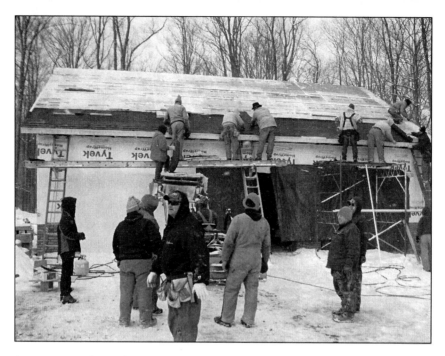

J.T.'s co-workers lay shingles after a snowfall, just one of many weather challenges they faced during scramble to finish the garage.

Allegheny Power employees: Tim Saxman and Tony Messina. In an interview with the local newspaper that publicized the good deed, Messina related how he told his boss it would be nice to complete the job started by J.T. almost three years earlier. Saxman replied, "Let's do it."

Allegheny Power employees from fifty-two service centers in three states pitched in with donations or labor. Local restaurants donated food to the volunteer crew, upwards of twenty-five people at a time. At one point, workers had to sweep four inches of new snow off the roof just to complete shingling. But they were determined to have a finished product before the family returned.

"It was so emotional just to see that," Marie-Paule said. "People we don't even know did this. It just blows your mind. It's just another beautiful story that shows a lot of people are good."

J.T. echoed her thoughts. "It made me feel people cared. I knew they cared. I don't need a building like that to know they care, but I know people want to do something with the situation we're in. I know nobody did this for publicity. It was all pure heart and friendship."

And then it was on to the business of life. Chad went back to school for only one day when he began vomiting. Although doctors had stopped his chemotherapy permanently, his parents had decided to begin giving him supplements and vitamins based on research they had done. Their first reaction was that the new pills might be upsetting Chad's stomach.

He also began complaining of new vision problems. When J.T. took him to their ophthalmologist, the physician said, "Chad's view is changing. He'll need new glasses."

Marie-Paule thought, *Ahh, it's only a change in the vision.* In fact, that night, when J.T.'s supervisor visited, he, too, was grateful the glasses had fixed the problem. "He just needed new glasses? Great! Our prayers were answered."

A few days later, however, Chad's vision deteriorated further, leading Marie-Paule to begin questioning her faith. "One day you think your prayers are answered, and now you're thinking 'no, they're not.' And it's those moments that kind of shake your faith. And you ask all those questions: Did we pray wrong? Did we do something that our faith wasn't strong enough? Where did we do something wrong? Not as God's punishment, but in the way I prayed and in my faith."

Chad vomited daily for the next two weeks, preventing him from returning to school. In addition, Dr. Hemminger had recommended he have an IV port installed in his chest, but the Scanlons weren't convinced it was necessary. Then one day at Hemminger's office, Marie-Paule asked the doctor's secretary, "Why do they want to put the port in him, for medicine or chemo?"

In a soothing voice, she said, "Later on he'll need medi-

cine, and it'll be so much easier. It's more of a comfort procedure than a major surgery. No one will see it; no one will
know it's there. If he needs it, it's there. It'll be so much easier on him."

So the port was installed.

Chad settled back into life at home just before Easter. His
condition continued to worsen. Between throwing up and
not eating, he kept losing weight. He also spent much of his
day sleeping on the couch.

Marie-Paule grew so concerned she phoned Muriel
Costello, who had once told her of a priest renowned for his
healing abilities. "Could you find the priest you mentioned to
me once and tell me who he is? I think we should try. There's
nothing else but the power of God for him, and I feel I need
to do something."

Mrs. Costello contacted the priest in Boston, told him of
the urgency in Chad's case, and set up a meeting for three
days later. She told Marie-Paule, "Everything's arranged.
You'll have a private audience to talk to him. He's already
praying for Chad."

Marie-Paule thought, *Great! We're going to see that priest.
Maybe this was meant to be. This is the answer. He's going to be fine.*

Mrs. Costello arranged for a jet to pick up the Scanlons
at nearby Latrobe Airport. Less than two hours later, they
landed near Boston and were driven to the priest's residence.
His house was modest. At the door, the family was met by
his housekeeper. "We're expecting you."

Inside, they met Father Celeste and several other people.
He then said mass, at one point laying hands on Chad's head
and asking God to "remove his tumor." Afterward, he asked
Chad, "Feeling okay? Sometimes healing happens quickly,
sometimes a little a day. It's not me healing, but God."

For those present, it was hard not to be moved by the
spirituality or the setting. Father Celeste had file cabinets
filled with cases of people who'd had unexplained healings.
He even gave Marie-Paule and J.T. oil for the sick to anoint

Chad with each night. It had a comforting aroma. Marie-Paule felt "lots of positive energy" in the room. Moreover, Chad finally rediscovered his appetite and ate as much pizza as he could.

Maybe that's it, Marie-Paule thought, *the beginning of a better time.* She remembers feeling like mothers in the Bible bringing a child for Jesus to heal. *I'm bringing Chad to Jesus who works through Father Celeste to heal him.*

On the flight home, Chad was so weary he rested on Marie-Paule's shoulder. His day wouldn't be over, however, until he greeted relatives arriving from Belgium later that night. His aunt and uncle, Madelyn and Paul, had one son, Jacques, and had recently given birth to a daughter, Bethany. She had been born on the same date Chad was discharged from The Children's Institute, and he desperately wanted to hold her for the first time.

It was Holy Week, and the Scanlon house was filled with friends and relatives, from near and far.

At times, Marie-Paule remembers, life that week bordered on chaos. "There were usually too many people in the house. The phone was always ringing; Chad was tired. On Easter Sunday, he spent much of the time on the couch, even though all the other kids were outside on an Easter egg hunt."

Following Easter, they took Chad for an MRI, partly to see if the homeopathic treatments were helping. Instead, they learned that water was accumulating around Chad's brain. The next morning, Dr. Hemminger called. "We need to put a shunt, or drain, in Chad's skull."

"Is it really necessary?" Marie-Paule asked. "What's it going to do?"

"For one, it should make him feel better. The fluid is probably causing all the nausea and vomiting." Then she added, "In addition, it might give him an extra couple weeks."

J.T. and Marie-Paule agonized over making Chad undergo yet another procedure. Marie-Paule was so overwhelmed with their situation she finally allowed herself to cry—and then cry some more. Before they made a final decision about the shunt, they returned to Children's Hospital to meet Debra Nicolette, a hospice nurse beloved for helping families adjust to the stark realities of a child's life-threatening illness. In a later newspaper interview, Nicolette said, "I am not the death nurse. I don't tell parents, 'Let's talk about how your child is going to die.' It's more like, 'What can I do to get you through this?'"

That day, staffers at Children's made a plaster cast of Chad's handprint, as a future keepsake for his parents. The gesture is routinely done when a child has been deemed terminally ill. Marie-Paule appreciated the sentiment, but not the circumstances. "Chad was too tired to even know what they were doing, first off. Second, they see this handprint as a story of a child's life . . ." She shakes her head. " . . . But the casting is still in the box they gave to us, sitting in his room. I looked at it once, but I just can't see his life in his hand. I know it's his hand when I look at it, and just want to grab and hold it. But I didn't like the way or idea of how it was done. It's not like a birth footprint. I see plaster, I don't think of his life. Instead, I think of the moment they made it because there was no more hope."

When the Scanlons returned home, Dr. Hemminger called to see if they'd decided on implanting the shunt. "The tumor's growing," she reminded them.

"Can you explain the procedure in a simple way?" Marie-Paule asked.

Hemminger said the fluid building around Chad's skull had nowhere to go, and was likely causing Chad's nausea and lack of appetite. By putting in the shunt, she explained, the fluid would drain from his skull into his stomach and be absorbed or expelled naturally. "He needs to have this drain, but you need to do it immediately."

Meanwhile, Marie-Paule's family was still visiting. Sasha was back in school. And now they had another medical crisis to deal with. In short, there were many balls floating in the air. "We managed," Marie-Paule says, "but it was difficult for all of us."

She continues, "When we went for surgery, it was scheduled for Thursday evening. He was supposed to be operated on, stay overnight, and come home the next day. We waited and waited, and eventually got a little upset. We told the nurses, 'Chad's not doing well at all, and he needs a bed.' So they brought us a bed and blankets . . . Later, a surgeon came out and said she might have to postpone the surgery altogether. Then she came back and told us maybe they could do it after all. So we thought, 'Great.' But after even more time passed, she finally came out and said they needed to cancel, telling us Chad was first on the list tomorrow, when he'd have a new surgeon who was well-rested."

The Scanlons were led to a small room with one bed for Chad. The stress of the day and thought of another surgery had frayed his nerves, his mother realized. "Chad, you're not talking."

"No."

"Are you scared?"

"Yes."

"It's okay to be scared. Are you afraid to die, or afraid of surgery, or both?"

He didn't answer.

"Chad, you cannot give up. You cannot give up hope. You still have to hope for a miracle. The doctor won't be able to do anything for you, but God can. He's the only one. We have to hope with all our heart." His mother steeled herself for what she was about to say next. "But at this point, I cannot lie to you, and say you are going to have a miracle. We still have to hope, still have to pray, but either way you will be healed, in heaven or here. Things will be better for you."

"I know Mom." He hugged her, and fell asleep in her arms.

The following morning, Chaplain Roger Jamison visited Chad while he waited for surgery along with nearly a dozen other children. He sang a religious children's song to Chad, which helped him relax. And when Chad went into surgery, Jamison took some time to talk with Marie-Paule.

She told him, "I guess I can't keep telling God what to do. I have to stop fighting and instead give it all to Him. Accept whatever's going to happen. I've spent too much time fighting God, because I'm not going to win the fight anyway."

"What, you're not one of those Christians who knows all the answers?"

"No."

"Me either."

Chad eventually came out of surgery. The surgeon told his parents, "Everything went fine. The fluid drained right away when I installed the shunt. We're taking an x-ray now just to be sure everything's still fine, but he'll be back in his room shortly."

In the waiting room, J.T. and Marie-Paule saw another Latrobe family whose son was waiting for an x-ray. He also had cancer, and was still walking on his own at that point. In the next several weeks, however, his condition deteriorated so rapidly he died.

Meanwhile, when Chad awoke in his recovery room, his parents noticed an immediate improvement. "Mom, I feel hungry." And when a nurse asked him to smile, he somehow managed, especially when doctors agreed he could be discharged that day.

When he returned home, he asked his Aunt Abby to make chicken noodle soup, which she did. He had hoped to watch Sasha play volleyball that afternoon, but never felt up to it. Instead, several of his fellow jump-ropers and their coach brought Chinese food back to his house. He talked with everyone for hours.

Chad's next few weeks were modestly upbeat as his appetite returned and his energy levels improved somewhat. For instance, in a Holy Trinity "marathon" fund-raiser, he walked a lap around the oval stadium track, followed by another in a wheelchair. He also planted flowers with his mother, then a peach tree, and even took a ride on a four-wheeler.

But even these activities fatigued him. He was also having trouble seeing well, and normally needed an arm to rest on just to walk. But not the day his dad came home one afternoon. Chad shuffled unassisted up the sidewalk thirty feet or so to greet him. "You made my day, buddy," J.T. said.

One of the more remarkable events happened in early May, not long after Marie-Paule's family had returned to Belgium. A fellow parishioner at St. Boniface Church offered to arrange an intimate prayer service at the Scanlons the fol-

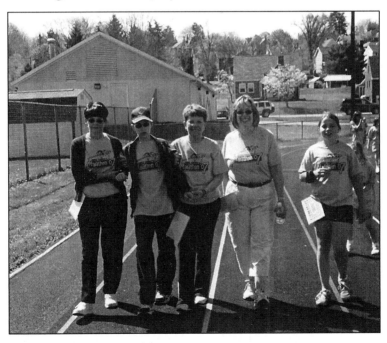

Chad with Sasha and his teachers at the Holy Trinity Marathon in Ligonier.

lowing Sunday after the 9 a.m. mass. "It'll just be whoever wants to come from church," she said.

During the week, however, word of the impromptu service spread to Holy Trinity School and beyond. Marie-Paule's biggest fear was that she might have to feed everyone who showed up. As it turned out, she would've needed to multiply loaves and fishes if that were the case. What started out as a few dozen grew to upwards of three hundred. That gorgeous spring morning, friends, family and people who barely knew the Scanlons parked in their ten-acre lawn and began streaming down the hill overlooking their house. To the pastor and lay people assembled on the porch to conduct the service, the scene was straight out of the Bible. A minister greeted everyone, and then two people read from Scripture. A few short prayers were read by others, and then the entire

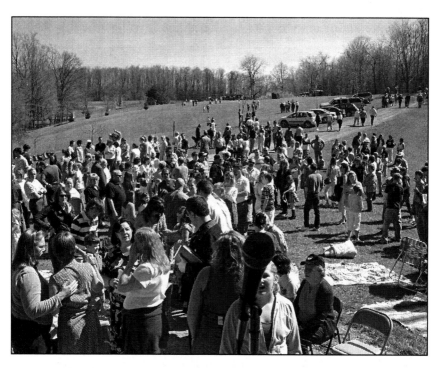

Impromptu prayer service at the Scanlon house after Easter 2007. Friends, family, and people who barely knew the Scanlons showed up en masse.

"congregation" joined in for a concluding prayer on Chad's behalf.

Marie-Paule summed it up this way: "All those different branches of Christianity coming there for one child, for the same reason, at the same place, praying to the same God. What's the difference, really? It was all the same faith."

In early May, two of Marie-Paule's relatives from Belgium flew in for a visit on very short notice. The couple was not particularly religious at that point, but instead comforted the family in practical ways. Marie-Paule says, "We didn't have to entertain them, or cook for them, or take care of them. Instead, they took care of us. They did the cooking and cleaning, and they slept in our unfinished basement because there was no room upstairs."

She continues, "Henri and Anne didn't go to church, but they were very impressed with Chad and our faith, that we took time each evening to hold hands and pray. They joined us every time; didn't seem to mind coming and doing it. And when they went home, they started praying with their kids, because being here was something they said they'll never forget. They came up with their own little prayer they say in Belgium as a family."

On the day the couple left, Chad had plans to attend an annual school fund-raiser where he used to buy flowers for his mother to plant in her garden. So he rested in the morning, ate lunch at home, and went with his mother to school in the afternoon. Numerous booths had been set up, and at one, he paid to throw a cream pie at a teacher. His classmates howled with laughter. Afterward, he asked to visit his classroom, so his mother took him upstairs. He sat in his desk. She sensed he was troubled. "What are you thinking, Chad?"

"I just feel that I've been cheated."

"Why?"

"Because all the kids in my class got to do a project about a European country, and I didn't. Sasha was supposed to help *me*, but she had to do all the work because I was sick. So I didn't learn anything." He looked at his mother. "Next time, I'm going to ask my teacher if I can do a project on my own." Chad went on to say he couldn't wait to be in seventh grade next fall. Then he and his mother went back to the bazaar, where he bought his flowers and a wooden fruit crate. Somehow each year he managed to buy the "perfect" gift for his mother.

When they left and went outside, a student's mother from Colombia approached and asked if she could pray over Chad.

"Oh. Okay," Marie-Paule said.

So the woman put her hands on him and began praying—in Spanish. "It was bizarre. I wish I knew what she said," Marie-Paule says—especially after what happened later that evening.

They eventually returned home. Chad took a rest in his bed while his mother folded laundry. When she came in later to check on him, he was trying to get up, but was in a terrible state. He had vomited and soiled himself, and his eyes were rolled back in his head. Marie-Paule called her mother and Sasha for help. She was convinced he'd had a seizure. She helped him stand, and then led him into the bathroom so she could clean him.

Without being asked, Sasha and her girlfriend cleaned Chad's bedroom. Marie-Paule knew she had to call the hospice service for help, but she had her hands full with Chad. She decided to call her friend Aurora, who managed to make the call for her. J.T.'s brother Bob also showed up, and carried Chad from the bathroom to the couch. Meanwhile, J.T. had to be called to come home.

When he arrived, she told him, "It's not a good evening to try and reach hospice."

"Why?"

"Rochelle, the nurse we like so much, is away celebrating her anniversary."

"What about other nurses?"

"Apparently, those on call are dealing with other hospice patients who've died, so we're just going to have to wait." But every time the front door opened that night, it was never a nurse. Friends and family kept showing up, leading her to say at one point, "If you are not a nurse, stay in or out, but don't come in and out. I want a nurse."

Later on, a hospice nurse did arrive, gave Chad some medication, and spent considerable time consulting on the phone. Afterward, she left. The following morning another nurse arrived. By then, Chad had stabilized enough to drink a bit and even try to speak.

In her mind, Marie-Paule thought he might be getting a little better. But as time went by, it was obvious he wasn't coming back, even though he was trying. She thought, *Maybe he just needs therapy, someone to teach him to speak, or massage his legs.* "But I was just fooling myself, I guess. I just wanted to see what I wanted."

By Sunday, word had reached Rochelle, who cut short her weekend getaway with her husband and rushed to the Scanlons' home.

She came by day and was relieved at night by nurses who gave J.T. and Marie-Paule a chance to rest. The whole family was sleeping in their son's room at that point. Chad and Marie-Paule on his bed, Sasha and J.T. on the floor, with the nurse nearby on a chair.

Within several days, Marie-Paule and J.T. had learned how to care for Chad on their own, and the overnight hospice visits ceased. At that point, they also arranged for a hospital bed that they moved into their bedroom so the family could sleep more comfortably together.

That's when Marie-Paule's friend told her she knew of three musicians who were willing to come and play for Chad. She thought he might enjoy the entertainment since Chad had played the violin as a boy and one of the musicians was a fiddler.

The trio came and performed several times at the house,

the second occasion in Chad's bedroom.

That was where I found them in late May. It was as sur-
real an experience as I ever expect to encounter. Three men
playing bluegrass songs for a dying boy. And yet that day it
felt perfectly natural.

Since Chad could no longer speak, he communicated by
gesture: Thumb up or down; two hand squeezes for 'yes,' one
for 'no.'

Oh, and one other gesture. During a lull in the entertainment, Marie-Paule said, "Chad, show everybody how we let
Daddy know when he's getting on our nerves." Eyes closed,
Chad lifted his right hand off the hospital bed and raised his
middle finger. Everyone in the room burst into laughter—
especially J.T.

But when the last song was played, Ray, something of a
guitar-playing minister, opened a Bible and read from James
5:13-14: "Is anyone among you in trouble? He should pray.
Is anyone happy?—"

Chad raised his right arm again, in affirmation.

"—He should sing praises. Is there anyone who is sick?
He should send for the church elders, who will pray for him
and rub olive oil on him in the name of the Lord."

The following week, I and several other friends offered to
spend a night at Chad's bedside to help his parents manage
a few minutes of uninterrupted sleep. However, J.T. called
the night before I said I'd come over. "We appreciate the
offer, Rich, but we think we've got things covered for now."

"No problem, buddy."

As it turned out, J.T.'s brother Blake took up a vigil one
of those nights with Chad. He was the only one awake as J.T.
and Marie-Paule were lying in their bed, as close as they
could be to their son.

By now, Chad was even having trouble communicating
with gestures. So when he awoke in the middle of the night,

Blake wasn't sure what was troubling him. At first, he presumed Chad was thirsty. He raised his nephew's bed to the sitting position and got the eyedropper out, just as his brother had done all week. But something convinced him water wasn't what Chad needed. Roused by the exchange, J.T. woke. "What's wrong?" he asked Blake.

"I don't know. Chad's awake but I can't figure out what he wants."

"Let me try."

J.T. came to Chad's bed, and lay down with him.

"Is something wrong, buddy?" he whispered.

Chad nodded his head slightly. His father moved closer to him and grasped his hand.

"Are you scared?"

Chad nodded.

J.T. studied his face intently for a few moments.

Then, in the quiet of the room, he said in a hushed voice, "Your recovery isn't going the way we hoped, buddy . . . It's okay to die, Chad . . . It's okay . . . Heaven is a beautiful place, and we'll all die, so don't be scared. Mom and I will be here with you now and some day in the future . . . It's okay."

Blake couldn't help overhearing J.T.'s words, which made an indelible impression on him. He would later say, "The exchange between father and son was so powerful. I truly felt God's presence. That night, I realized a young boy and his parents would get through the very worst circumstance imaginable."

By Friday afternoon, May 25, I hadn't heard from anyone. I decided to make an unannounced visit. When I got there, I met a subdued group of Scanlon relatives on the front porch, which struck me as perfectly natural. "How's he doing?" I asked J.T.'s brother.

He looked surprised.

"Rich, Chad passed a little while ago."

Chad's passing marked the end of his young life but not the conclusion of his story. Just the first few chapters in many respects. Months after his funeral, Marie-Paule and J.T. decided to establish a charitable foundation in his memory. The Chad Delier Scanlon Memorial Fund supports causes he championed: physical fitness, learning and helping others in need. Within months of its inception, the fund raised $67,000 from generous donors.

The Scanlons also agreed to be interviewed for this book about Chad, partly to keep his memory alive and partly to offer solace to other families who are forced to cope with life-threatening illnesses. Rather than make it a how-to guide, we decided to chronicle Chad's illness as best they remembered it. If readers want inspiration on how to cope with life's ultimate challenge, they will find abundant examples of how he and those who loved him dealt with his illness.

And finally, all proceeds from this book will go directly to Chad's fund (www.chadscanlonfund.com), which is under the umbrella of the Community Foundation of Westmoreland County.

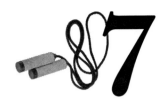

Memories

Years ago, there was a Scanlon family reunion at Chad's grandfather's house. It was a large affair attended by aunts, uncles, cousins and their offspring.

I remember seeing Chad, who was only three or four years old at the time, walking all by himself down by the old barn, which stood along a dirt road away from the party. He was crying, the tears obvious from a distance because his boyish face was so dusty.

Anyway, they were real tears and I felt bad for Chad because he was obviously upset about something, but I couldn't understand what was making him cry. Then it finally dawned on me—the reason I couldn't tell was because Chad was crying in French. I did a double take because the Scanlon clan is composed of Irish-American, English-speaking folks. As far as I know, none of us speaks a second language. And here is this poor, pathetic, bilingual child crying in French.

I stayed with Chad until he found his mom, who scooped him up in her arms and offered him the comfort, understanding, and love that made everything better for him.

I'll never forget that the first bilingual Scanlon was that crying little boy.

—*John Scanlon, cousin*

Memories of Chad come to me in powerful snippets. They summon heartfelt emotions to the surface and make me miss him over and over. I remember Chad, Sasha, and my daughter, Amy, the three of them inseparable, riding in the back seat of our car to jump rope demonstrations, singing to Disney songs. Amy would do a high-pitched imitation of one of the lead singers and they would all laugh. They'd make Amy's stuffed snake "snakey poo" come over the seat and say rude, funny things to me. "Bad snakey poo." They often looked for some hidden spot after practice just to be together, talk and laugh. I can picture Amy and Chad jumping together, pairs partners, the chemistry between them so inspiring. He would treat her like he was her big brother, teasing her when they were working through a routine, coming up with nicknames for her and each member of the team, even me—"Coachy-Poo." I remember how Chad and Amy would both support each other when things didn't go well and how they'd cheer each other on through a hard workout or a competition event. After his last regional tournament, Chad wore all his gold medals around his neck. We took team pictures and started for home. A little further down the highway we met at the same rest area in Ohio and Chad was still wearing his medals. His Dad was joking with him that it was probably time to take them off. He smiled but kept them on, so proud of all he'd accomplished.

Chad's compassion for others was way beyond his years. He had a special understanding about how his friends were feeling. If one of his teammates was upset, he was right by her side. When the team was in New Orleans for the Junior Olympics, Chad was the first person to think of getting a gift for a fellow jumper who couldn't be with us. He took the lead with his compassion and others would follow.

I remember him teaching Christian how to swim in the hotel swimming pool. Chad offered to pay Christian a quarter if he could swim one lap across the pool. That was all the motivation he needed.   Christian made it and Chad handed him the coin.

There were so many good memories during Chad's last year: Walking with him for ice cream from The Children's Institute. Demonstrating for the patients at the Institute the night Chad was able to go home. We were all filled with so much hope for his recovery. Watching him demonstrate at the Pittsburgh Heart Walk, just nine weeks after his surgery. He was overjoyed to be jumping the team routine.

There are also painful memories: Sitting next to Chad at the edge of the pool at The Children's Institute talking about how many post cards he was receiving. He told me how much he had wanted to be a cartographer when he grew up; now he feared he wouldn't be able to do that. I told him never to give up on his dreams, but he was quiet. He seemed to be preparing himself for what was to come.

I can see him stroking his mother's hair. It seemed to bring him so much comfort and a peaceful moment between the two of them. I'll never forget the phone call after his last MRI telling me that the cancer was back. All I could do was tell him how much I loved him. It was so inadequate, not the cure that he deserved. I felt such horrible, gut-wrenching helplessness.

Then there was holding his hand in the middle of the night while Marie-Paule, J.T. and Sasha slept. That last night I was with him, he looked at me in the dark and was so restless. I felt like he wanted to tell me something but couldn't speak. So we "spoke" to each other with our eyes, shared the peace of the night, and continued holding hands.

The memories keep coming. And I keep missing him. Some days, it feels like he's in our midst watching us, smiling at us. Other days he feels so far away. My faith tells me he's in a spectacular place with God, but my heart wishes he was right here, where my memories keep him close. But that feels like a mere drop of water in the midst of an unquenchable thirst.

—*Laurie Whitsel, jump rope coach*

My eight-year-old daughter, Michaela, and Chad became fast friends in second grade. With his help, she was quickly accepted by their fellow students her first year at Holy Trinity. The same year, Chad's beloved grandmother, Helen, died from ALS. While at one of the viewing sessions at the funeral home, Chad and Michaela went for a walk outside. There was a graveyard next to the funeral home, and they walked in that direction. The sun was setting, and grief and sadness lay heavy in their hearts. Chad mentioned how well his grandmother had dealt with her impending death and how she had tried to help everyone else though it. He said he thought he could never go through what his grandmother had with such amazing grace and strength.

As the two talked about death, they both hoped and promised that they would never have to leave each other before it was time—meaning when they were "old and gray." Michaela then said, "What would you do if God wanted you before that time?"

"If that's what God wanted, I would do His will."

Years later, when Michaela and Chad were on the jump rope team, he fell ill the Friday before the Holy Trinity High Flyers were scheduled to compete in Junior Olympics. Knowing he had been diagnosed with a brain tumor, his teammates went to the competition with heavy hearts. But even then he didn't fail them. Only a few days after his brain surgery, he was calling them all with words of praise for how they'd performed at Junior Olympics. My daughter, Emily, was especially tickled by his compliments.

But that was just his way—supporting and cheering his friends even when he himself couldn't participate. Late in his illness, when he couldn't walk without help, he still managed to yell "Go, Michaela!" as she prepared to serve in a volley-ball game. That touched her deeply.

So I think it's safe to say Chad was wrong when he thought years ago that his strength and courage in the face of death couldn't compare to his grandmother's. Truthfully, his amazing grace and calm inspired us all, just as it would have his grandmother.

The person Chad was lives on in all his teammates, classmates, friends and family. He is here, with us all, and continues on with us through life.

—Mary Long, family friend

After Chad became ill, all of his friends and relatives tried to do whatever they could for his family: cooking suppers, washing laundry, or just being available. One day, after leaving their house, my husband Greg said, "I want to do something just for Chad."

So he called his friend Bernie Patrick, and asked if he would come play fiddle music for a friend's sick son. He told him about Chad's illness. Bernie said, "Just set up a time and I'll be there."

Bernie came one afternoon with his brother and another musician, and they played for Chad. He smiled and smiled, and seemed to be enjoying the performance so much. Just being there, watching him, made us realize that no matter what was going on in our lives, family and friends are more important than anything else—so spend as much time with them as you can.

Marie-Paule and J.T. lost their child, and Marie-Paule her best friend. No matter what, Chad thought of them first, and especially wanted to make sure his sister Sasha was okay. During Chad's illness, the Scanlons became a stronger family than they ever were.

And just remember, my friends: he will be with you, in your hearts and souls, always.

—Charlotte Goodman, family friend

My brother and I did a lot together. Yes, we did have our moments when we fought. But through everything we always stuck together. For instance, when we were living in our family's trailer we slept in the same room. Chad couldn't wait until we moved into the new house, because he always wanted his own bedroom. He used to say, "No one would go into my room but mom."

But it didn't last. Even when we moved into the house, Chad and I slept in each other's rooms like it was a sleepover. We also practiced jump rope together down in our basement. But I'll never forget this one time when Chad woke up in the middle of the night and went to my parents' room. He told them," I don't feel good." And then he threw up all over the hardwood floors. It went everywhere!

Mom and dad took care of him and cleaned up the mess. However, since we do everything together, it was my turn. An hour or so later, I went into my parents room and said, "I don't feel good." Then I threw up all over the floor my parents had just cleaned from my brother's mess. That was one night with Chad I'll never forget.

As Chad's 12th birthday approached, he was sick and still in ICU. He had always wanted an iPod. He would talk about having one, what music he would put on it, and what color he might get. He had to explain to my parents what an iPod does and how it works. He knew how expensive they were but that didn't stop my brother from dreaming.

So I thought I would get Chad an iPod for his birthday and put some music on it that would calm him, maybe help him sleep. One day, after visiting Chad in the hospital, I went home with Mrs. Whitsel, our jump rope coach, and she took me to Best Buy to get Chad's present. I shouldn't take all the credit, because Mrs. Whitsel actually paid for it. But she told me that it was from me.

The next day, I went back to my Uncle Sam and Aunt Molly's house, (where I usually stayed) and asked my expert uncle to help me. He told me that I could go to work with him the following day and use his office to put music on Chad's iPod. I went to work with him and all of his employees gave me CD's to put onto it. One of them, Tonya, took me to Wal-Mart and picked out speakers with me. We also got this "iDog," which moved and danced with the music it was playing and changed colors.

The next day Uncle Sam took me to see Chad, like he did every day, and I went into the room with my parents. I said hi to Chad, talked for a little bit, and then asked what he wanted for his birthday. "What I want is too expensive for you; you wouldn't be able to afford it.

"Tell me anyway."

"An iPod."

"Here you go."

He couldn't put ear buds in so we put some soft music on for him.

He was so happy it was unbelievable. I felt like the best sister in the world.

I miss Chad very much and I will never forget him. Not one day goes by that I don't think about my brother.

—Sasha Scanlon, sister

Charismatic (Billy)

One thing that really shined about Chad was the way he never complained about his sickness. When we went to Stations of the Cross, a kid in the class said, "My knees are killing me." Instead of saying, "Stop complaining and look what I am going through," Chad said, "You shouldn't complain; Christ went through great pain because he loves us." I cannot forget that.

Heart Warming (Marc)

Chad always had a way of making people smile, whether it was a joke or a silly game. I really liked when he was explaining the joke about the snail. Chad was his own person, and made his own choices. He could have played baseball or football but he picked jump rope and he did not care what people thought about that. He was just happy with himself.

Amenable (Autumn)

My favorite memory is when Chad and I were walking back from Saint Boniface Bible Camp. We saw this black thing on the road and we thought it was a snake. We ran the whole way back to the church and we explained what we'd seen to Father Simon. He drove us home and on the way he stopped to pick up the "snake." It ended up being a piece of rope. We had a good laugh every time we thought of that funny day.

Delightful (Joshua)

One day, on Chad's birthday, Aunt Marie-Paule planned a scavenger hunt. Chad had to make the teams and he picked me. It made me feel happy, cared for and not left behind. Chad was very thoughtful not to leave people behind.

(Aunt Anne)

It was in July 1998, and Chad and Sasha were at Bible school. At noon I went with Marie-Paule to pick them up. In the van, both of them were really happy and talkative. It was a hot sunny day and the windows were wide open. Chad put his head out and started to sing: "Glo-o-o-o-o-ria in excelsis deo" with all his heart and all his voice. It was so funny, his joy was so deep! Thanks, Chad for the fresh air of Christmas in July.

(Uncle Bob)

How Chad my nephew,
How missed thou are.
Your smile and laughter
Like a shining star

So young, so strong
You jumped your rope
with all your heart.
Here we are, many months later.
wondering what happened …
You are known for being caring
and I know with time
we'll get our bearings.
Writing these words hurt so clearly
with my love, so dearly.

—Uncle Bob, Aunt Anne;
cousins Joshua, Marc, Autumn and Billy

As we drive up over the Ridge
Someday we'd like to build a bridge
To the void up in the sky
Where the little boy went to die.

Though his life did not go far
He was so much like a shooting star
So quick and bright throughout the night
So brave and strong throughout his fight.

We know he is in a happy place
Because we can still see his face
We know he is here in our heart
Because we will never be apart.

But now it's time to say goodbye
To that little boy up in the sky
Someday we'd love to see him again
To fulfill the happy end.

—Cousins Josh, Zack, Breanna, Patrick, Morgan,
Uncle Ben and Aunt Heather Scanlon

My parents used to say that Chad and I knew each other before we were born. I guess you could say that's true, because our parents met years ago in birthing class while our mothers were pregnant. This may have had something to do with why we became best friends, but I think that God had planned for us to be best friends even before birthing class.

When we were about three, we started preschool together at the YMCA. We became closer and closer ever since. After "graduating" from pre-school, we began attending Holy Trinity School together.

In kindergarten, we became almost inseparable; we literally spent every waking moment together at school. I remember at naptime our sleeping mats were always beside each other's. Even outside of school we spent bunches of time together. I remember going over to his house and eating dinner with his family, which was always entertaining for me. And each winter, Chad, my dad, and I would spend a day and go down to Pittsburgh. Wherever we went, if we went to the zoo, the aviary, or even the incline plane, we would always have a good time.

Chad was gentle, kind, caring, funny and most of all my best friend. He would do anything for me, even stand up against the "big, bad Mrs. Farabaugh." You see, when we were in first grade we had to start learning how to take AR tests on the computer, which back then was in Mrs. Farabaugh's room. At times she may appear to have a tough exterior, but deep down she is a very kind and caring person. But when I was seven, it was very hard to look past the tough exterior, and I scared easily. Chad, on the other hand, wasn't afraid of her. (Well, even if he was, he never showed it.) So, when the day came that I had to take my AR test, Chad willingly offered to come up with me. So together, we made it through.

He was a good student, an amazing athlete, and a great musician. And even if he wasn't any of those things I wouldn't have cared, because what really mattered to me was that he was a true friend. I truly miss him.

—*Rachel Chattaway, classmate*

The first time I saw Chad after his surgery, I have to admit I was a little nervous. I didn't know what to expect. I walked to The Children's Institute where he was undergoing rehab and went directly to the reception desk to find out how to get to Chad's room. The next thing I know I was being hugged from behind. When I turned around there was Chad. I couldn't believe my eyes. I thought we would find him confined to bed. Not only was he standing there, but we also went outside for a long walk. Chad made me feel so comfortable. His strength was endless, and we had a great visit.

But my fondest memory of Chad was on Secretary's Day in April 2007. He wasn't doing well, and was the last person I expected to talk to. I answered the phone in the school office to hear, "Happy Secretary's Day, Mrs.Flickinger."

"Thank you, but who is this?"

"It's me, Chad. I just called to tell you to have a great Secretary's Day."

I was speechless. When it finally hit me that the caller was Chad, I was so touched by his act of kindness that I will never forget that day. In fact, every Secretary's Day for the rest of my life I will imagine his voice saying "Happy Secretary's Day, Mrs. Flickinger." It will always make me smile for being one of the lucky ones who knew him.

—*Debby Flickinger, secretary*

One day when I was at Chad's, we decided to go for a walk. We walked about one mile down the hill to a stream. We were looking in the water when we saw a palomino trout. It was huge! We were excited and determined to catch it. We didn't have fishing poles with us so we decided to try and catch it with our hands. We went into the stream and tried and tried to catch that palomino—laughing and having a great time—when I fell into the water and got soaked.

Chad began laughing and said, "Oh shit!" Actually, we both ended up pretty wet, and after about fifteen minutes we still had not caught the palomino. Wet and cold, we headed back up the hill through the woods to Chad's house. We carried on the whole way until we got so cold we called his dad for a ride.

When we got back to Chad's I had to borrow clothes of his to wear home. It was a day I will never forget. Chad was my best friend and the only one that ever really understood me. I miss him very much.

—*Dominick Shawley, friend*

It still hurts to think of Chad in the past tense, but as time moves on certain memories of him bring a smile to my face. I recently found a poem Chad had written about me in English class. It stated that I was a friend and a Penn State fan. This triggered another memory that shows Chad's character. The first day he came to school after his surgery, he told me that he would have worn his Penn State shirt except he didn't have a dress down pass. How many people do you know that under the circumstances would still follow the rules?

Chad was a great student, and he was normally very self disciplined. One day when I was reading "A Tale of Despereaux" to his English class, something tickled his funny bone. He started to giggle uncontrollably. Next, the rest of the class started to laugh at Chad, and we all ended up in hysterics.

In 2008 we dedicated our yearbook to Chad. This year as his class graduates, my editors, Rachel Chattaway and Michaela Long, again wanted to do something special for him. From the moment this decision was made, it was like we were guided by Chad. We thought we might do something with the celestial star that was named after him. So we looked through a clip art book, and right in front of us was a picture frame with stars in our school colors, blue and gold. Our next job was to find a Bible verse to coordinate our ideas. I Googled "Bible verses—stars" and the first verse to pop up was just what we wanted. We think we had help on this page.

I think of Chad every day and smile. He will always be in our hearts. I know that Chad knows all of the answers to the questions we used to discuss in Bible study. I hope to discuss these questions further with him someday.

—*Connie Beam, teacher*

This is a story about Chad, Jimmy and Marie-Paule that I thought I might never tell any one. Chad's cancer was far advanced. He was days from dying. Whenever I was around him, I prayed for his relief and comforted him as best I could. I was already starting to miss him.

I was watching Chad a few hours so his parents could rest. It was very late this particular night. J.T. and Marie-Paule were lying in their bed, as close as they could be to Chad. I was imagining what was going through their heads as they tried to sleep, or if they had even had a single hour of sleep in the last twenty four.

Chad couldn't speak and could barely communicate with hand or body motions. Nevertheless, because he was so smart, he could get his point across—at least to his parents. In fact, he may have communicated the strongest message I have ever witnessed.

I was watching him when he seemed to indicate he was thirsty. I raised his bed to the sitting position and got the eye dropper out, just as his father had done all week. But he convinced me this wasn't what he needed. I tried all the obvious remedies but he still needed something else. Finally, Jimmy woke up, came over, and laid down with Chad

"Is something wrong, buddy?"

Chad nodded his head slightly. Jimmy laid a little closer to him and held his hand.

"Are you scared?"

Chad shook his head "yes." Jimmy studied his face intently for a few moments.

Then, in the quiet of that room, he whispered, "Your recovery isn't going the way we hoped, buddy . . . It's okay to die, Chad . . . It's okay . . . Heaven is a beautiful place, and we'll all die, so don't be scared. Mom and I will be here with you now and some day in the future . . . It's okay."

I was in tears, but Jimmy remained strong, and Chad needed that. He felt that confidence when he needed it most. Jimmy comforted his son, and Chad's acceptance gave his father some peace that night.

The exchange between them was so powerful. I truly felt God's presence. That night, I realized a young boy and his parents would get through the very worst circumstance imaginable.

—*Sam Scanlon, uncle*

I received a call from Jimmy on July 16, 2006. At the time, we had Allegheny Power crews working in Philadelphia on storm trouble. He told me his son had experienced a bad headache and was now in UPMC, and that he needed to take a vacation day.

When I got off of the phone, I called our crews together in Philadelphia and said a prayer for the family. After we returned to Latrobe, all of the managers kept in contact with me for updates on their situation. Then the email network took over and grew between all fifty-two service centers and power houses. At this point all I really knew about the Scanlon family was that Jimmy had a wife named Marie-Paule, a son Chad, and a daughter named Sasha.

One day, a lineman came up with the idea to finish building their garage. We had no budget, but with the touch of a button sending out emails, the money started rolling in. I'll never forget the sunny day when we started: we had to use torpedo heaters under the roof to melt off the snow so we could put the shingles on. Volunteers showed up from many service centers. Some knew each other, some didn't; and some were not even particularly fond of one other. But we all worked side by side for a common cause. I could feel Chad's love for his family there, giving us strength and determination to get the garage finished before the Scanlons returned from their trip to Hawaii, courtesy of the Make-a-Wish foundation.

My relationship began as Jimmy's supervisor, but it grew to becoming friends and ultimately being referred to as "Uncle" Tom. I never believed Chad would leave us, or lead me on the most amazing, yet heart-wrenching journey of my life. I would learn and watch how Chad and his family dealt with each trip to the hospital, and each return home. To watch and talk with Chad was such a rollercoaster ride. Just when we thought all was going well, he would have another setback. But during all of the many trips back and forth to the hospital, Chad's faith shined through. When I went to watch him practice with his jump rope team, he looked so strong and happy, not like a boy who was battling brain cancer and fighting for his life. I just knew all our prayers were going to be answered and Chad would beat the odds.

I was given a rubber memorial bracelet at the Holy Trinity School prayer service for Chad. This bracelet was a source of hope and love for Chad. I still wear this bracelet today, because it still gives me hope for the future.

I sometimes look at my bracelet or look at the pictures we took with the Scanlon family, and thank God for bringing Chad into my life, if only for a short time. Even now, when my wife Mary and I go to visit, or stop by to say hello, I can feel Chad's presence. I don't think that will ever change, nor do I want it to.

In early May of 2007 we heard about a prayer service that was being arranged for Chad at the Scanlon's house. It was a beautiful spring morning when Mary and I pulled into the lane and parked. We walked towards the house with many other friends and family members. Hundreds of people would eventually make their way to the service, surrounding the house. You could just feel the love and positive energy.

When the readings and prayers and music were finished, Chad stood up from his chair and with help from his Dad, thanked everyone for coming. Jimmy motioned for Mary and I to come and say something to Chad, so we went forward. Chad thanked Mary for making lasagna and sending it over a few days earlier. He said it was the best lasagna he had ever eaten.

We left that day with tears blurring our vision as we drove home in silence. All I could think of was how this 12-year-old boy could have the grace and love and kindness to thank Mary for some lasagna—while he was fighting the battle of his life. If anyone I have ever known deserved a miracle, he did. I was still hopeful he was going to get one.

The next time we came to the house, Chad was bedfast and resting in his parent's bedroom. We didn't know what to say or do for Marie-Paule and Jimmy. So we gave Chad what would be our last hug and kiss, told him we loved him and wished him peace.

This extraordinary family amplifies courage, hope, love and inspiration. They have two children: one is earning her wings, and the other is wearing his.

—*"Uncle" Tom and "Aunt" Mary Waltz, friends*

Recovering from his first surgery, Chad slowly awakened. Taking time to gather his wits, he wanted only to feel the soothing affect of water on his lips. A few minutes later he tried to talk but couldn't. He labored to overcome the tubes and the effects of the anesthetic. As he struggled, the first words out of his mouth were, "Dad, thanks for not letting me die." What twelve year old would be more concerned with thankful praise toward his parents than asking for something to drink or make the pain go away? Anyone who has been operated on knows that when you wake up your lips are dry and all you want is a drink of water.

Although Chad's earthly time was short, his impact was timeless. We remember him not because he is gone, but because he touched all of us. This young man faced death, yet he never struggled. He experienced pain, yet never complained. He faced God and accepted him freely.

I remember a story told to me by J.T. He and Marie Paule wanted to put Chad on an organic food diet with no sugars. They tried it for a while but Chad didn't want to comply. One day, J.T. was trying to convince Chad that the organic diet may help. While walking up the driveway, J.T. asked him, "Do you see that plastic jug sitting their alongside the driveway?"

"Yes."

"If I told you that eating it would cure your disease, would you eat it?"

"No Dad. If God is ready to take me, I am ready to go!"

During a sermon at church a priest told the following story. A teacher distributes a box to each of her students. She tells them that in this box is the greatest thing God ever created. Of course they open their boxes and dump out the contents. A super ball and candy bar fall out. The kids are baffled. The teacher reaffirms that the greatest thing God ever created is in the box. The kids, questioning this, look into the box and see a mirror at the bottom. They see their reflection and realize, "I am the greatest thing God ever created."

Chad was the greatest thing God ever created.

—*Art Scanlon, uncle*

It was a beautiful spring day in western Pennsylvania. The sun was shining and there was a spring chill in the air. We decided to take a ride and visit the Scanlons. On our way, we noticed they were fishing at Grandma Weaver's swimming hole. We stopped, parked the car and went to visit them.

There had been a storm a few weeks back and a tree had fallen across the creek, so Marie-Paule, Heather and I climbed onto the tree and sat and watched Jimmy, Uncle Dale and the kids fish for a couple of hours. At the end of the fishing excursion, I bet Chad five dollars he wouldn't jump into the creek. That kid stripped to his skivvies and jumped straight into the water! Let me tell you, that water was cold. So naturally he got out with blue lips, chattering teeth and asked for his five bucks. I hate losing a bet but I paid off this one with a smile on my face.

I will never forget Chad's mischievous smile and that look in his eye as he said, "Aunt Amy, you owe me five dollars." To this day, I don't know what he bought but if I were to take a guess, it would have been an ABBA CD. His love for adventure and music are only a few of the wonderful qualities he had. There isn't a day that goes by that I don't think of Chad. I just thank God that this is just one of many wonderful memories that I have of my nephew.

—*Amy Scanlon, aunt*

When Chad was just a toddler, my wife Helen would carry him outside at night and show him the stars. One night there was a full moon, and she pointed to it as she explained what it was. For the longest time, he called her Mooney. We couldn't figure out how he came up with that name till someone remembered her showing him the moon.

I remember one day I was splitting firewood across the road in the parking lot. There was snow on the ground. At that time, Jim and Marie Paule were living in a trailer, near where I was working. Marie-Paule wanted to send me a message so she wrote it down on paper, dressed Chad up in nice warm winter cloths and boots and sent him out to give it to me. When I finally got the message, I took him by the hand and followed his tracks back to the trailer. It reminded me of that little boy in the comic strip called the Family Circus. What should have been about a fifty-yard walk wound up being two-hundred-fifty yards. He walked over and watched the creek flow out of the pipe under the road. He walked over and looked over the bank and pushed snow over it in several places. He walked around about three different trees and made two circles around my burn barrel.

I should have known then that this was a child with a very curious mind—that he would eventually be interested in history, birds and fish. He was curious about everything he came into contact with.

His sense of humor was also very sharp. He called me the Cookie Monster because he knew my love for cookies. One time I was taking a nap on the couch when I woke up and there was a cookie on my stomach. When I asked him how that cookie got there, he gave me that wry grin of his and said, "I'll never tell."

These are just some of the many things I'll always remember about Chad. You couldn't help but love him.

—*James Scanlon, grandfather*

I remember going rafting the summer before Chad was diagnosed. It was 2006, and we had gone to my Pap Pap's house to visit. My little sister was afraid and didn't want to go so Chad took her place. I remember going over the rapids, "falling out" and swimming. We even went down one rapid on our behinds. As I think back now I wish we could still have great times together.

I think it was unfair that Chad had to go so soon. My grandma had died just four years earlier, and now my cousin had died and I would never see him again. It was terrible. I was at a baseball game the night he died. My dad had to leave in the middle of it to calm down my sister. When we finally got home and he told me I just went and sat down and tried to not believe it—Chad couldn't have gone. He was so kind and caring and I couldn't just accept that he was gone. I sat there for over an hour doing nothing.

My mom came out and talked to me. She told my sisters and me that Chad didn't deserve to go. That he would always be with us even if he couldn't talk to us anymore. I remember that and think how Chad tried his best at everything and no one stood in his way. He went to the Junior Olympics for jump rope, and was an altar server at his church. He was so good that I can't think why God wanted him in heaven. Now two years later I don't know how I got through it. I don't think I would have if it hadn't been for my parents but most of all, God. I prayed to him every night and he led me through it. Now I'm in high school and I am still not happy about it but I have grown to accept that there is nothing I can do but pray for Uncle Jimmy, Aunt Marie-Paule, and Sasha and hope they get better.

—*Blake Partlow, cousin.*

All my brothers and sisters met at my brother Art's house in New York for his son's high school graduation. I remember Chad had a headache. I thought to myself, how could an eleven year old have so many headaches?

Well, it wasn't long after that visit that we got the call that Chad was in the hospital and was seriously ill. I couldn't believe it. Our entire family pulled together to try to find out what the best treatment was for him. We all did research on the computer looking for that miracle cure, but we just couldn't find anything that would make a difference. All we could do was hope and pray that they could get rid of the cancer in his brain. As I tucked my own children into bed every night, I thanked God they were healthy, and prayed that God could cure Chad.

Then one morning tragedy struck my family. We were in a car accident and two of my daughters were seriously hurt. My oldest daughter, Sami, had some internal injuries, broken bones, and eye problems. They were serious but not as serious as Chad's. My middle daughter, Alex, had a traumatic brain injury. She was in very serious condition.

I realized how fast life could change in just a split second. One moment you are getting ready for a party, laughing, joking and having a good time; or you are going to school to help out with a project and suddenly—life changes.

My oldest daughter, Sami, got released from the hospital after four days. I was still in the hospital with my other daughter, Alex. I had no idea what my daughter would be like when she came out of her coma. I remember Jimmy called me and was sorry that he couldn't come and be with us. Here you are with your own child who is dying and you want to help me. I told Jimmy that he had enough to worry about. Just keep us in your prayers and we will still keep Chad in our prayers.

I would talk to Marie-Paule and we would compare notes on Chad and Alex's therapy. She would tell me things that

Chad was doing in therapy and I would tell her things Alex was doing. We shared a common bond and it was nice to be able to talk to someone who was going through something similar.

There was a major difference though. Every day that Alex would wake up, I would see a major improvement. I would live for mornings because she would improve so much with just a good night's sleep. My heart would fill with more and more joy.

On Marie Paule and Jimmy's end, their hearts would get heavier and heavier with worry and sadness. Chad would get worse and worse and there was no cure for him.

Why does one person receive the miracle of life but another does not? Does it make us stronger? Does it make our faith stronger? No one will ever know why children have to die. It just doesn't seem fair. How does God pick and choose?

I remember the last time we saw Chad alive. I pulled the kids from school and we headed home to Pennsylvania. It was a day of mixed emotions for them. They were happy to be out of school, but anxious and nervous to see Chad. My children knew that he was going to die. It was a beautiful spring day in April and we sat out on the porch and he told us all about his trip to Hawaii. It was good to see him and joke with him.

Jimmy and Marie Paule are two of the greatest parents I know. They showed love the entire time Chad was sick. They opened their home to everyone, and they never gave up.

—Aunt Audrey Partlow

One evening, I prepared a meal to take to the Scanlon's house to share with them. I hoped I could keep my emotions in check. Chad knew he wasn't going to recover.

As we settled down to eat, I was nearly moved to tears. What greater gift could there be, but a family still enjoying the simple gift of a meal together? Would I be so gracious if this was my family's situation? Would I welcome friends into my life even when the end of time becomes evident?

Rather than become emotional, I smiled, and rejoined the conversation, now aware of the gift I was receiving, both from the Scanlons and from God. As dinner ended, the evening continued outside, around a campfire where more family stopped by to visit. We talked and laughed as Sasha played with her dog and Chad snuggled by the warmth of the fire that his dad built. Meanwhile, his mom lovingly wrapped him tightly in a blanket to hide him from the cool evening air. Later, as we were leaving, Chad told us his favorite joke, as we lingered by the door and he rallied his strength and joy to entertain us all. Precious time, special moments, togetherness unmatched by any other, recorded forever in our hearts.

Chad and his family taught me valuable lessons. To allow others to share time and life with you is a personal and significant gift. Welcoming them into your heart to love and nurture you is a two-fold reward. Putting on an appearance of strength, independence, and self-sufficiency means denying others the opportunity to help you, to share time, to nurture, and to really care for you. Thinking that I was giving to the Scanlons was my mistake. It was their invitation to their family circle and savor their precious time together that was the purest act of giving. I am forever grateful to them for the gift, and for sharing their family and dear Chad with me and so many others.

—Barbara Glista, friend

While I was driving to see Chad at the hospital after his brain surgery, I was overwhelmed with so many emotions—sorrow, frustration, anger, even my own weakness. I wasn't sure how I was going to handle seeing him face to face.

At the hospital, we talked for a while about jump roping and school. He was still disoriented and tired from his surgery, and his vision was impaired. But somehow he managed to stay awake for all his visitors.

Nonetheless, I was scared for him, and frustrated how this could happen to someone so young. It was hard to muster the right words to say. In that moment I felt weak. But not Chad; he seemed so strong.

As I got up to leave, I remember him rising out of bed to walk me to the elevator. I was so surprised that he wanted to do this in his condition. He showed me that day that he was a young man of extraordinary qualities and that he was brave and full of life. He showed me the strength and courage that people only talk about. He never talked about life being unfair or complained about it. He shared his life to the fullest and showed others how to do the same. Chad made me look at life differently and I am proud to have been his godfather.

—*Casey Olczak*

When I think of Chad I smile, right away, and it lasts for a while. The first seconds of my smile are intensely happy, with sweet thoughts of him because he was such an amazing kid and made a really big impression on me. But as my smile continues, I feel sad because of what he had to go through, and all that happened, and I usually shake my head to myself. Then, my smile grows wider because I envision my favorite memory of Chad.

As his former case manager at The Children's Institute, I

was blessed to meet and form friendships with Chad's sister Sasha, Marie-Paule and J.T. Once Chad was discharged, he began coming back for outpatient therapy. The whole family came to visit me when he arrived for an appointment. Usually I was in my office, and they would come into the hallway laughing and smiling and we would hug and catch up. Then they would usually make fun of me in some way or another about the work I was (or wasn't) doing. They liked to tease me about being too serious.

So imagine my surprise when I came back from a meeting and walked into my office to find Chad sitting in my chair, leaning back, his feet on my desk . . . smiling. I'll never forget that.

—*Becky Gloninger, The Children's Institute*

I routinely refer kids to the Make-A-Wish Foundation and talk to their staff at least once a week. So I wasn't all that surprised when they called to tell me Chad had gone on a trip to Hawaii for his wish. However, my contact then said that he had only been given about a month to live. " I wouldn't even have called," she explained, "but when you referred Chad, I could tell by the way you talked that he was really special to you."

That's the best way I could describe Chad—special. Despite all that he was going through, he always had a smile and loved joking around with his family and our staff. He truly enjoyed life and exuded a joyfulness that is hard to capture in words.

I keep a picture of Chad on my bulletin board at work. He is in the snow wearing a bathing suit, his arms flung wide and a look of pure joy on his face. The photo makes me smile every time I see it, and it reminds me to embrace the small joys in life as Chad always did.

—*Christine Meier, The Children's Institute*

Over the course of my career as a speech therapist I have treated hundreds if not thousands of kids with terrible brain traumas, some for up to a year. Chad was my patient in The Children's Institute hospital for less than three weeks, and yet knowing him has had a most profound and lasting effect on me. From the moment I met him I knew he was an extraordinary person, mature way beyond his years. He remained incredibly positive about his situation, never complained and continued to work hard to get better. His parents were a model for him in those respects. He took joy in his many interests and accomplishments and readily shared that joy with everyone around him. Even though he was tired, in pain and confused the first day I met him, he told great stories. His smile was infectious.

It was Chad's sense of humor that connected us most, I think, along with our "nerdiness," which I mean as a great compliment. We both collected postcards that we began exchanging as soon as he started to go home for visits. He gave me one from a town in Belgium, the pronunciation of which I butchered (sort of on purpose to give him a giggle). He never let me forget that and he teased me mercilessly, continuing to make us both laugh. When I sent him a card from vacation telling him how I got lost in the woods and had to call 911, it was the same thing. His timing with a joke was impeccable for a young kid. Although he took great pleasure in making fun of me he was always somehow kind and respectful about it.

The last time I saw Chad was at his house just two weeks before he passed away. He was too weak to sit up and had to be on the couch in the living room while his family and visitors sat at the table. Every once in a while I'd hear a weak chuckle from him after I'd spewed some nonsense. There he was appreciating silliness and enjoying his life up until his much too premature end. What an inspiration. I miss laughing with him.

—*Sue Hersh, The Children's Institute*

My best memory of Chad is his love for being challenged. I met Chad several days after his surgery at Children's Hospital, and continued to work with him during inpatient rehab and outpatient rehab. From the first day I worked with Chad I could tell that he wanted to be pushed and looked forward to conquering the challenges that lay ahead of him.

On that first day of therapy Chad was eager to get out of bed and get moving. He had little awareness of his left side and was requiring quite a bit of assistance getting dressed and ready for the day. Chad was eager to tell me that he was on a jump rope team and that he would like to get back to this activity. While brushing his teeth he needed me to give cues for him to remember to brush the left side of his mouth. All of a sudden he began speaking in French and the thought ran through my head was "there is much more to this kid than meets the eye." Over the next few weeks and months I grew to understand that Chad's rich experiences as a child had shaped the person he had become. He didn't back down from the challenge that he had been dealt, and his family's support helped to give him the strength to continue to face the challenges he met on a daily basis as he resumed his daily activities.

Chad loved playing games that challenged him mentally and visually during therapy. He took these activities into his home and school, to share his experiences in rehabilitation with friends and family. Chad made incredible gains in a short time in therapy, largely due to his willingness to try, and sometimes fail, in order to make gains in the end. I continue to tell Chad's story to my patients as inspiration, yet words alone can't fully describe who Chad was as a person and character he had that helped him through the challenges that life handed him.

—Ken Reichl, The Children's Institute

In the summer of 2005, J.T., Marie-Paule, Chad, and Sasha came to visit us in New Hampshire. This particular day we took a walk through the woods and ended up by the small brook that runs near the road we live on. Since it was a nice day, we decided to spend some time at the brook and wade in the water. I wasn't about to go in the water because the day before we saw a monster of a crayfish in it. This crayfish was so big it looked like a lobster. But that didn't deter Chad from going in. First he took off his shoes and started in the water. Then his shirt came off. It only took a few more minutes before we saw Chad lying in this cold mountain water where the "Killer Crayfish" lived! When I reminded him about the crayfish we saw, he said he would go look for it...and he did! I am happy to say that he never did find that crayfish, and to this day we have never seen it again. Every summer when I take the kids for a walk and we end up at this same brook to play in, I share this story of Chad with them. They will always remember him as I do—a smart, happy, and extremely caring young man.

—Aunt Laurie Wilkinson

One thing for sure, Chad, we didn't get to know you enough. We had the chance to spend some time together when you and your family came to visit in Belgium and also when we came to see you in the USA. That week will stay forever in our hearts and minds. We came to you thinking, "It might be the last time we are going to see or talk to you," but deep down we didn't want to believe it. We hoped to the end you were going to be okay somehow.

Even so, you remained the same nice, gentle joker, always in a good mood, the little polite boy. Despite your disease you blew us all away: never mad, never a word louder than another, yet you had every right. It was a real joy to spend time with you and to be there to support you. We never felt so much happiness and suffering at the same time.

We will remember each and every moment spent with you: like the time your courage allowed you to go outside and show us your peach trees, and the time we planted flowers together. Your willingness to please others and make people happy was stronger than your suffering itself. You changed our lives. You allowed us to understand what life is all about; that love for family is stronger than anything. Despite all that, we had to let you go. Your life was an inspiration we will never stop talking about.

—*Nicolas and Marie Delier, Belgian friends*

It was Christmas 2006 and all I was hearing was news of Chad through conversations on the phone. He was diagnosed in July and I could not take being away from him anymore. I had to come and see for myself if he was okay. I needed to see my grandson.

Being almost 80 years old, I wasn't very comfortable traveling by myself, so Marie-Paule and J.T.'s Belgian friend offered to be my traveling companion. She also wanted to be there with them. After spending about two weeks with my daughter's family, I was reassured about Chad's condition. He looked amazingly well and I was happy to be going home to tell everybody.

Before leaving, we had our last meal together, and that day Chad gave me a little gift. He then asked me a couple of times, very quietly, "Please mamie, don't go, stay." I told him, "I'll be back Chad, I promise." Chad's gift was a little Willow Tree Angel. I went home and set it up where I could see it all the time. After Chad left us for a new life, I picked up my angel and took a close look at it. I didn't know those

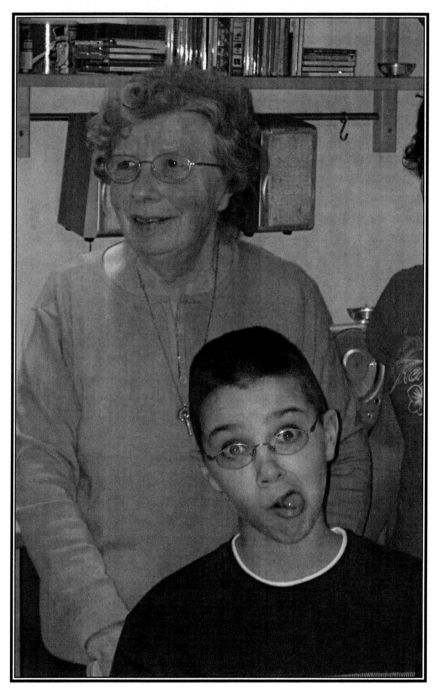

Chad acting like a goofball with his grandmother "Mommy the Belgique" from Belgium.

angels had names. My angel's name is Love Simple Pure. Thank you, Chad, for that little angel watching over my home. What a sweet idea it was.

—*Madeline Destrebecq, grandmother*

Marie-Paule was the first person to trust me with the life of a godchild when, at the time, life didn't see fit to give me one. I could not dream of a better godson than Chad. He was incredibly caring towards everyone. He was also very curious. Learning was a pleasure for him.

Eventually, I had my first child, Simon. And on July 22, 2006, he answered the phone call from my sister Anne in the U.S. I was five months pregnant with my second child at the time. I was worried because the call was coming so early in our morning. Anne told me Chad was life flighted, that he had bleeding in the brain. All kinds of thoughts started to run through my mind: my daughter Lucie would be born soon and her cousin Chad was fighting for his life.

Nevertheless, Chad was an optimistic child. He was passionate about living and following surgery promised me to get out of rehab the day Lucie would come. As it turned out, she was born August 18, the same day Chad did come home. In Belgium, we celebrated Saint Helen's Day (also the name of Chad's deceased grandmother).

We came to visit for Easter with my mother. Chad wasn't well; he was sleeping a lot and didn't have any appetite. I was sitting by him with Lucie on my lap when he asked me to help him cut his food. He opened his arm to hold Lucie and my eyes filled up with tears. Chad, Lucie, and I; no others witnessed this unique moment.

We were supposed to stay for two weeks. Every evening we would pray as a family with Chad. I could tell that the end of our stay was going to be difficult. But airport delays on the East coast of the United States gave us an extra three to four days. When I went to tell Chad about it, he said, "I know, I asked God in my prayers for you stay longer." Those extra days were a blessing for us because Chad was feeling a little better.

Chad, to whom I felt so close, will always be some sort of an enigma. I often wonder what his future would have been. He was capable of great things. So why did he die when he had such strong faith? He is not here to live the rest of his story, so it is up to us to keep his spirit alive.

—*Francette Delier, aunt and godmother*

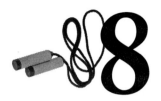

Epilogue

Marie-Paule Scanlon, October 2008: "I still think God could've healed Chad the way we wanted. Why he didn't I don't know, and that's why I struggle. But it doesn't make me believe that all those stories in the Bible are just stories. I still believe He heals people, that miracles happen. Why not with Chad, that's just my big question. I sometimes wonder if my faith was strong enough, or if I didn't understand my Bible the right way. But why would God do that to Chad if it's my fault, not Chad's? So that's what I don't understand. But if it had to happen again, I would just pray as hard as I could.

Post Script, May 18, 2010: In one week, it will be three years since Chad passed. Two days ago, J.T. and I met with Chad's former oncologist and the president of Children's Hospital to finalize last-minute details in this book, which will go into print shortly.

When the doctor asked how we were coping with losing Chad, I basically reiterated what I said above: We just didn't get the miracle we were hoping for.

"But you did," she said. "Your miracle was that he awoke from the coma following his surgery. None of us, including the surgeon, was sure he would ever wake up . . . we thought the brain damage was just that severe. At the time, I was wondering why I would even treat the brain tumor of a boy who might be in a vegetative state."

I was stunned. After Chad had his emergency surgery, I thought he had been heavily sedated so his brain could heal, not realizing he was actually in a coma from which he might never have regained consciousness. The doctor was right; God had given us our miracle—a chance to have ten more precious months with Chad, time to prepare, and time to say good-bye.

I know we will see Chad again some day and it definitely helps me to go on. Also, knowing that he helped a lot of people by bravely handling his illness makes me realize all this pain wasn't in vain."

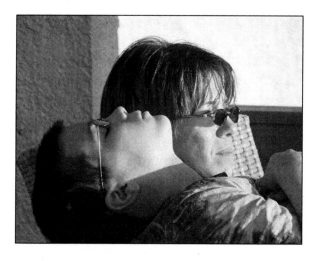

Chad and Marie-Paule relaxing in the sun on the balcony in Hawaii during his Make-A-Wish trip

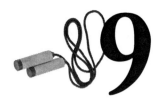

Acknowledgments

There are so many thanks we need to extend it would probably take another book to list them. First we thank the good Lord for giving us the privilege of creating and raising two wonderful children, Chad and Sasha. Although the time with Chad was shorter than expected, the twelve years He gave us with him were exceptional.

There was so much moral, physical and spiritual support from the time Chad was operated on until the moment he took his last breath. Thank you to all of our family and friends who helped us through the most difficult times of our lives. People cooked many dinners for us, they visited on a continual basis, they constructed a garage for us while we were on a Make-a-Wish trip to Hawaii, and they prayed hard for us and we believe they still do. This group of people is much too large to mention by name because the list would stretch around the world. There were soldiers in the Middle East fighting a war who took the time to send Chad a post card or a gift. One solder even sent him a scarf from Afghanistan to give to Marie-Paule for Christmas. It amazes us how much good there is in a world of negativity, and a smile is in our hearts thinking of the things you all have done for us.

To the United Bowhunters of Pennsylvania we send our sincere appreciation for the hunt you sent Chad on in North

Carolina. We wish we had video capturing his excitement when he harvested those two deer. Like MasterCard, it was priceless. Thanks also to your members who sent Chad gifts for hunting and accepted us into your club, and gave Chad a bow and taught him how to shoot it.

Holy Trinity School did everything possible to accommodate Chad with his school work, while granting Marie-Paule time off to take him to his doctor appointments and take care of Sasha.

We would also like to thank three women at Magee Hospital who catered to Chad when he was going through a difficult MRI due to headaches. They adopted him as their "little brother" and showed him so much love and affection in this difficult time.

To the doctors who worked on Chad at the emergency room at Excela's Latrobe Hospital: your quick diagnosis and actions gave us another blessed ten months with him. To the doctors at Children's Hospital who operated on Chad with great precision: we all expected some sort of mental handicaps from the operation and the only problem he encountered was the left field of vision. A job well done. To Chad's oncologist, we express much gratitude. The start of our relationship was rocky. You were the giver of bad news all the time and we were always nervous to see you but you and your staff turned out to be a great support team for us. We know you didn't like the outcome of Chad's situation and didn't want to believe it but thank you for your guidance. You along with the hospital chaplain helped us spiritually cope with Chad's outcome.

The Children's Institute was a special place. It was there we saw the greatest healing process in Chad's ordeal. We witnessed him recover to the son we knew.

The Make-a-Wish Foundation receives special thanks also. They planned and delivered Chad's Hawaii trip without a flaw. This memorable getaway helped us escape the reality of life for one week. That time will be forever embedded in our minds.

—*Marie-Paule, Sasha, and Jim Scanlon*

LaVergne, TN USA
30 November 2010

206738LV00005B/156/P